PAEDIATRIC ULTRASOUND

Edited by

Helen M. L. Carty

MB BCh FRCR FRCPI FRCP (Lond) FRCPCH FFRRCSI (Hon)

Professor of Paediatric Radiology and Consultant Radiologist
Alder Hey Children's Hospital
Liverpool U.K.

Authors

Sharon F. Crawford, DCR(R), DMU, MSc
Superintendent Sonographer
Ultrasound Department
Alder Hey Children's Hospital
Liverpool U.K.

Julie B. Higham, DCR(R), PgDip
Senior Sonographer
Ultrasound Department
Alder Hey Children's Hospital
Liverpool U.K.

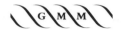

Visit our website at:
www.greenwich-medical.co.uk

Distributed worldwide by Plymbridge Distributors Ltd

Typeset by Saxon Graphics Ltd, Derby
Printed in Spain by Grafos

CONTENTS

PREFACE

Children are not small adults. They have a different spectrum of disease in addition to those seen in adult medicine. This book on Paediatric Ultrasound has been written to provide an introduction to the techniques of sonography in children, and a brief synopsis of children's pathology which may be seen on ultrasound examination. Sonographers receive most of their training on adult patients but, when in clinical practice, are also asked to scan children. We hope this short book will assist them in this task.

H.M.L.C.
S.F.C.
J.B.H.
February 2001

ACKNOWLEDGEMENTS

We would like to acknowledge the generosity and help of colleagues in providing images.

1

PAEDIATRIC SONOGRAPHY

A child's perceptions and fears differ greatly from those of an adult. A frightened child is an uncooperative child. Time spent by the ultrasonographer in allaying fear and gaining cooperation is time well spent. The following advice and hints, we hope, will be useful.

Hospital environment

A welcoming, child-orientated environment will help to lower a child's anxiety level. The waiting area should be well lit and warm, decorated with pictures and posters and have a variety of suitable toys and books. Information displays about ultrasound examinations written in simple language help parents to explain the procedure to their children. Ideally children should have separate waiting areas from adults and be allowed to play.

The room

The ultrasound room should always be prepared prior to calling the patient. Speed, accuracy and timing play an important role in paediatrics. Initially, the room should be well lit with a dimmer switch for during the examination. The room should be kept at a suitable temperature and it is important to consider the needs of each individual; e.g. the temperature of the room may need to be raised when scanning a neonate.

There should be pictures, posters, mobiles and suitable toys, particularly musical toys, which can be used to distract the child during the examination.

Preparation of the patient

A leaflet clearly explaining the examination is essential. This should be written for the children in children's language and should include details of any preparation required (e.g. a full bladder) before their visit. If needed, flavoured fruit drinks should be given to the child in the department.

The ultrasound examination

Once the child and parents have entered the room and their details have been checked, a repeat explanation of the examination must be given. Asking them questions and also giving them the opportunity to ask you questions will help to establish a good rapport. Good communication and a cheerful, friendly atmosphere will help to lower a child's anxiety level and help to gain their trust in you. The examination is much easier to perform on a willing child but needs vary considerably with age. It is therefore important to be adaptable to all their requirements.

Neonates

Respond to eye contact and – some more than others – to noise. Handle gently and do not startle them with rough movements or cold jelly. Gentle soothing rubbing movements are settling.

After 6 months

Babies wriggle and grab at anything in sight, but most of all they want their mothers. Musical toys act as a good distraction in this age group.

Toddlers

This age group varies considerably, from the willing cooperative child to the hysterical screamer! When children of this age group are removed from their daily routine and surroundings they are prone to temper tantrums. They tend to be suspicious and apprehensive and it is important to reassure them that the examination is painless. Showing the child the equipment and letting them touch the gelled transducer will help to alleviate fear. Books and toys may aid in distracting the child during the scan. Parental cooperation and confidence is vital!

4–6 year olds

This group is generally cooperative. They should be directly spoken to in suitable language. They are becoming independent from their parents, especially whilst all is safe and well. However, when faced with unfamiliar surroundings or anticipated discomfort they can become devastated if their parents are not at hand. Reassurance, compliments and encouragement are often all that is required.

Over 7 years

Children are more independent and usually very cooperative. However, they can be troublesome and belligerent, particularly if they sense inexperience. They still need lots of encouragement and reassurance.

Adolescents

The requirements of adolescents vary, as this is often an insecure time with mood swings from independence to dependence, but they should be treated on a more adult level. They are often very self-conscious and embarrassed about their bodies, if they are asked to remove any clothing; it is therefore important to respect their privacy. A 15-year-old boy attending for an ultrasound examination of testes may prefer his parents to wait outside during the examination.

General tips

- Encourage parents or a familiar nurse to be present during the examination.

- Use distraction techniques. By encouraging the child to watch a mobile, play with a toy or even to count, you can perform the examination more easily. Timing, however, is important. Start too early and the child will lose interest; too late and they will pay no attention. Older children find an examination more interesting if shown the screen and the images are explained.

- For babies and young toddlers, dummies dipped in glycerine can be used to stop crying.

- Neonates and babies lose body heat quickly. Leave covering and clothing on until the last possible moment, then perform the examination with speed and accuracy.

- Remove the minimum of clothing consistent with the examination. Don't take off underwear if avoidable.

- Never insist that a child must lie down for a scan. Adapt your technique. It is easier to perform an examination on a willing subject even if they are not in the most ideal position.

- Always examine a non-painful limb or area first to allow the child to become accustomed to the probe.

- Always examine the bladder first when performing renal and abdominal examinations on babies, as they invariably empty their bladders when the gel is applied to their skin.

- If the bladder is very full and the child is distressed, scan the bladder first and let them empty it before continuing with the remainder of the examination.

- If the bladder is not full when scanning a neonate, carry on with the examination, as their bladders fill quite quickly, and re-scan it at the end.

- Cineloop facility is an invaluable tool, as often children do not lie still and find it difficult to hold their breath. It enables review of a few frames and a good image to be selected, rather than scanning for long periods, trying to freeze the image at an exact moment.

- If all else fails, bribery with the promise of a certificate and a badge will usually gain a child's cooperation.

The ultimate aim in paediatric sonography is to perform an ultrasound examination producing images which accurately depict normal/abnormal anatomy, but this should never be to the detriment of the child.

After the examination

After the examination the child should be happy and relaxed and rewarded with a certificate, pictures to colour and badges. Communication is again important. Pass on information about the scan and ensure parents know where to go for results, e.g. GP, clinic appointment.

2

THE HEAD

Due to its portability and ease of performance trans-fontanellar sonography remains the initial examination of choice in the identification of hydrocephalus and haemorrhage. The preferred method of imaging for many of the congenital anomalies, replacing ultra-sonography, is now MRI.

The patent anterior fontanelle is used as an acoustic window. Closure begins at about 9 months of age and is usually complete by about 15 months. This is there-fore a limiting factor.

PATIENT PREPARATION
None.

CHOICE OF TRANSDUCER
5 or 7 MHz curved transducer.

7 or 10 MHz linear for evaluating superficial structures such as the extracerebral spaces or cortex.

TECHNIQUE
Patient position: supine, the patient being wrapped in a sheet or blanket if required, to stop movement. The infant may lie in the long axis of the couch or trans-versely across it dependent on operator preference.

The patient's head is gently held in position (chin/cheeks) by parent or nurse.

The transducer is placed on the anterior fontanelle and angled to produce 5 or more images in coronal section, and rotated through 90 degrees and angled to produce three or more images in the sagittal plane.

Cross-sectional sonographic anatomy

Coronal sections (see Fig 2.1)

Coronal sections are obtained through 5 levels of the ventricles:

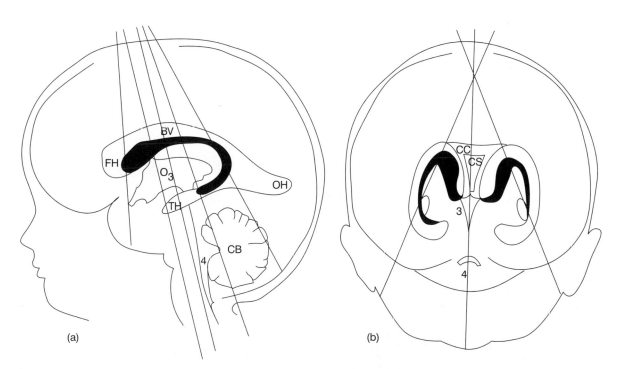

Figure 2.1 — Schematic representations of standard scanning planes: (a) coronal and (b) sagittal.

FH frontal horns
BV body of ventricle
OH occipital horn
TH temporal horn
CB cerebellum

3   third ventricle
4   fourth ventricle
CC corpus callosum
CS cavum septum pellucidi

1. Frontal horns anterior to the foramen of Monro
2. Foramen of Monro
3. Posterior aspect of the third ventricle through the thalami
4. Quadrigeminal cistern
5. Trigone of the lateral ventricles.

ULTRASOUND APPEARANCES

1. *Frontal horns* (Fig. 2.2) – anechoic paramedian fluid-filled spaces with a crescent shape configuration.

   The hypoechoic corpus callosum forms the roof of the frontal horns.

   The anechoic cavum septum pellucidum (CSP) forms the medial wall.

   The echogenic head of the caudate nucleus forms the lateral wall.

   Pulsations from the anterior and middle cerebral artery may be observed in the interhemispheric and sylvian fissures respectively.

   The frontal and temporal lobes appear hypoechoic.

2. *Foramen of Monro* – The lateral and third ventricle communicate through the foramen of Monro.

   Anechoic triangular CSP is seen between the frontal horns of the lateral ventricles (Fig. 2.3).

   Frontal horns of the lateral ventricles are fluid filled.

   Third ventricle can be seen as an echogenic structure beneath the CSP.

   Pons and medulla (brainstem) appear echogenic.

3. *Echogenic interhemispheric fissure* – seen midline (Fig. 2.4).

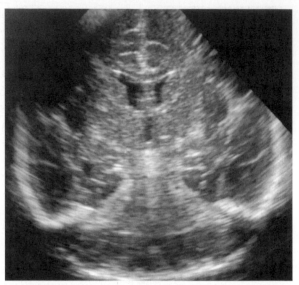

Figure 2.3 — Crescent shaped anechoic frontal horns, anechoic CSP, echogenic third ventricle, brainstem posteriorly.

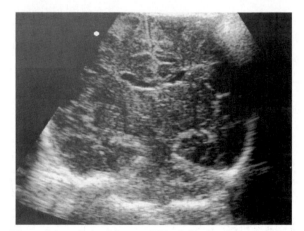

Figure 2.4 — Frontal horns, CSP, thalami, pons, cerebellum, echogenic interhemispheric, choroidal and Sylvian fissures.

   Anechoic frontal horns with anechoic CSP.

   The thalami are seen inferiorly to the CSP.

   Inferior to the thalami are the echogenic choroidal fissures.

   The tentorium appears highly echogenic.

   Pons and cerebellum are seen posteriorly.

4. *Quadrigeminal cistern* – echogenic and lies superior to the echogenic cerebellar tentorium (Fig. 2.5).

   The bodies of the lateral ventricles are seen superiorly and are bordered by the caudate nucleus and thalamus.

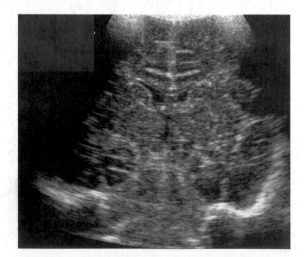

Figure 2.2 — Crescent shaped anechoic frontal horns, corpus callosum and CSP.

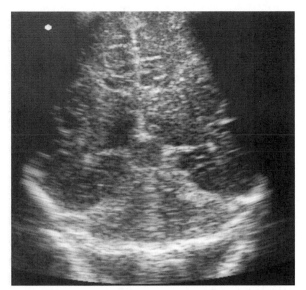

Figure 2.5 — Echogenic quadrigeminal cistern, echogenic cerebellum, body of lateral ventricle, thalamus.

5. *The lateral ventricles* diverge laterally (Fig. 2.6).

Within the trigone of the lateral ventricles is the highly echogenic choroid plexus.

Lateral to both trigones are normal areas of increased periventricular echogenicity.

Inferior to the ventricles is the echogenic V-shaped tentorium and cerebellum.

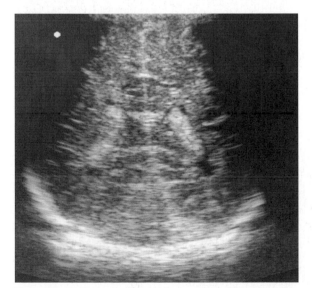

Figure 2.6 — Echogenic choroid plexus within the trigone of the lateral ventricle. Inferior to ventricles is V-shaped tentorium and cerebellum.

Sagittal sections

Planes are obtained through:

1. The midline.
2. The frontal horns and lateral ventricles.

ULTRASOUND APPEARANCES

1. *Midline* – CSP appears as a fluid-filled structure lying between the anterior horns of the lateral ventricles (Fig. 2.7).

Superior to the CSP is the thin, crescent-shaped corpus callosum.

Third ventricle is small, fluid-filled.

Inferiorly is the echogenic cerebellar vermis which is indented anteriorly by the triangular shaped fourth ventricle.

2. *The anatomical landmark* is the caudothalamic groove – a thin, echogenic band lying between the caudate nucleus anteriorly and the thalamus posteriorly (Fig. 2.8).

The caudate nucleus is normally slightly more echogenic than the thalamus.

In premature infants the germinal matrix is located immediately anterosuperiorly to the caudothalamic groove.

The highly echogenic choroid plexus in the trigone of the lateral ventricle is seen.

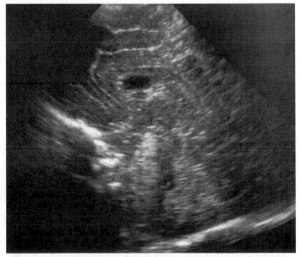

Figure 2.7 — Midline section showing crescent shaped corpus callosum, third ventricle and inferiorly the cerebellar vermis indented by the triangular shaped fourth ventricle.

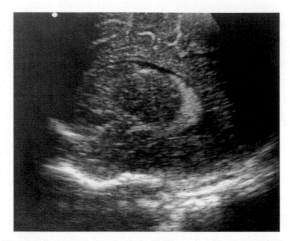

Figure 2.8 — Section through frontal horns and lateral ventricles showing caudothalamic groove, caudate nucleus and thalamus. Echogenic choroid plexus is seen in the trigone of the lateral ventricle. Note periventricular halo or blush.

The choroid plexus extends anteriorly into the body of the lateral ventricle and courses inferiorly into the third ventricle.

Normally the choroid plexus has a smooth contour.

The frontal, parietal, occipital and temporal lobes surround the lateral ventricles.

Posterior to the occipital horns, the normal area of increased echogenicity (periventricular halo or blush) can be seen.

Generally, images further lateral to the ventricles are not obtained as there are no major vascular or ventricular structures to act as landmarks.

A variable number of cerebral convolutions can be seen which increases with gestational age.

Sagittal sections can be useful to confirm an abnormality noted on coronal images.

Normal variants

Asymmetry of the lateral ventricles, particularly the occipital horns which are often larger than the frontal horns.

Ventricular size changes with maturity: with increasing fetal age the size of the lateral ventricles decreases relative to the size of the cerebral cortex. Thus the ventricles of the premature infant appear relatively larger than those of the term infant.

In the term infant the lateral ventricles, especially the frontal horns, may appear compressed or slit-like, reported in about 60% of normal subjects. This variation needs to be recognised when assessing the neonatal brain for the presence of cerebral oedema.

Slit-like ventricles occur in infants with cerebral oedema with other findings such as increased echogenicity of the parenchyma, poor definition of sulci and gyri, and decreased vascular pulsations.

Choroid plexus
Never extends into the frontal or occipital horns.

Lies within the body of the lateral ventricles and the temporal horn.

Is normally thin with a smooth outline.

Becomes bulbous in the region of the trigone where it forms the glomus.

Focal thickening in areas other than the glomus should arouse suspicion of haemorrhage.

Never extends beyond the caudothalamic groove.

Periventricular halo
Echogenic halo around the posterior part of the lateral ventricles in almost all normal neonates.

Present in full term infants but not as prominent.

The aetiology of the halo is unclear – could be related to the white matter fibres or could be a scanning artefact as it cannot be reproduced in all scan planes.

PITFALL
Must be distinguished from cerebral haemorrhage and periventricular leukomalacia.

Hydrocephalus (neonatal)

Hydrocephalus is a condition marked by an imbalance of CSF formation and absorption. The resultant excess of CSF within the central nervous system produces ventricular dilatation, an increase in intracranial pressure and compression and thinning of the brain substance. However, recent work challenges this traditional theory by suggesting that it is an alteration in the normal haemodynamics of cerebral circulation that affects CSF circulation.

Approximately 80–90% of normal CSF production is by the choroid plexus of the lateral, third and fourth ventricles. The remainder is from the ependyma and arachnoid.

Normal CSF flows from the lateral ventricles to the third and fourth ventricles before exiting the ventricular system through the foramina of Magendie and Luschka into the cisterna magna and the basal subarachnoid cisterns.

Hydrocephalus is

Obstructive – non communicating – in more than 90% of cases.

Non-obstructive – with communication.

Obstructive hydrocephalus

This is due to mechanical obstruction to CSF flow and is characterised as intraventricular or extraventricular.

Intraventricular

Obstruction within the ventricle is usually at:

Foramen of Monro

Aqueduct of Sylvius

Foramina of Magendie and Luschka.

Extraventricular

Obstruction can occur anywhere along the extraventricular path of CSF flow, or within the basal cisterns.

Non-obstructive hydrocephalus

Infrequently hydrocephalus is non-obstructive or dysfunctional and is usually related to increased CSF production from a choroid plexus papilloma.

CLINICAL PRESENTATION
Increasing head circumference, bulging fontanelle.

ULTRASOUND APPEARANCES
- The normal ventricular system of the head, which appears as anechoic fluid-filled space becomes dilated and increases in size.
- The most useful qualitative features of early ventricular dilatation are ballooning of the superolateral angles of the frontal horns (Fig. 2.9). These areas dilate more than the trigones and bodies of the ventricles because they are larger and require less pressure for distension.

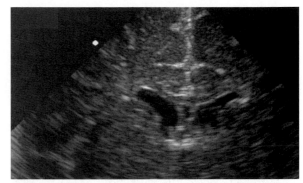

Figure 2.9 — Coronal section showing early ventricular dilatation; ballooning of the superolateral angles of the frontal horns.

- Depending on the stage of examination there may be multiple septae across the ventricular bodies with echogenic blood clot in the ventricles.
- The site of intraventricular hydrocephalus is identified as the point of transition from a dilated to non-dilated ventricle.
- If the foramen of Monro is obstructed there is lateral ventricular enlargement which may be asymmetrical.
- Aqueductal stenosis is associated with dilatation of the third and lateral ventricles; the fourth ventricle is normal or small (Fig. 2.10).
- Obstruction of the foramina of Magendie and Luschka produces cystic dilatation of the fourth ventricle and variable degrees of dilatation of the third and lateral ventricles (Fig. 2.11).
- In extraventricular obstructive hydrocephalus and dysfunctional or non-obstructive hydrocephalus there are dilated lateral and third ventricles and varying degrees of fourth ventricular dilatation.

CAUSES
Haemorrhage in the premature infant.

Meningitis.

Congenital malformation.

Haemorrhage

Echogenic blood clot obstructs the ventricular system. May be associated subdural collections.

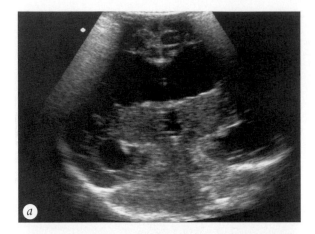

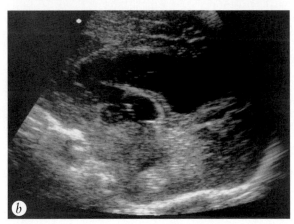

Figure 2.10 — Coronal (a) and sagittal (b) sections showing aqueductal stenosis, i.e. dilated third and lateral ventricles, normal fourth ventricle.

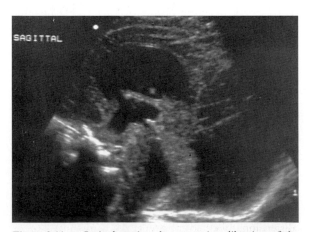

Figure 2.11 — Sagittal section demonstrating dilatation of the lateral third and fourth ventricles.

Meningitis

Debris in the ventricles. Measurements of ventricular size can be made using a ratio or index but direct visualisation of the entire ventricular system is usually adequate to provide a diagnosis of hydrocephalus.

The maximum diameter of the ventricles in the coronal and sagittal planes should be measured and recorded so that progress may be monitored (Fig. 2.12a, b).

TREATMENT

Drainage of CSF either by ventriculo-peritoneal shunt or third ventriculostomy.

Ultrasound can be used to document the position of the shunt catheter. Intracranial shunts are highly echogenic and easily recognisable (Fig. 2.13a, b).

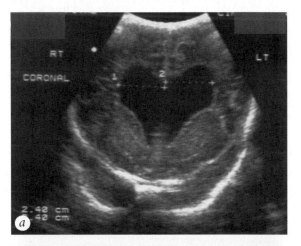

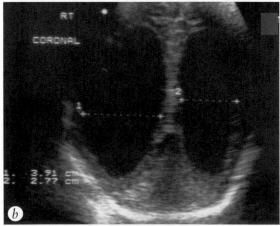

Figure 2.12 — Coronal sections showing measurement of (a) frontal and (b) lateral ventricles at their maximum diameter used to monitor progress.

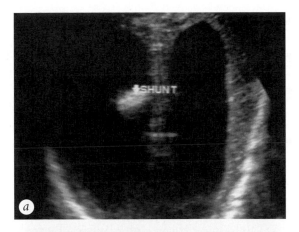

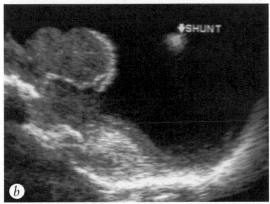

Figure 2.13 — Coronal (a) and sagittal (b) sections showing the echogenic intraventricular shunt tip of a ventriculo-peritoneal shunt system.

POST SHUNTING APPEARANCE

- Position of the echogenic intraventricular shunt tip should be noted and its relationship to the choroid plexus as this can get wrapped around the catheter and obstruct it.

- Large undrained loculi should also be identified and documented.

- Malfunction may also occur due to blockage of the lower end shunt tubing in the abdomen, usually due to infection. A CSF collection around the shunt tube is shown by ultrasound of the abdomen.

MERITS

Ultrasound can:

Confirm the presence or absence of ventricular dilatation.

Differentiate between obstructive and non-obstructive ventricular dilatation.

Identify the cause of hydrocephalus.

Ultrasound is also useful in follow-up evaluation of ventricular size in patients treated with insertion of a shunt system.

ASSOCIATED ANOMALIES

Chromosome abnormalities, e.g. Trisomy 13, 18 and 21.

Haemorrhage

Intracranial haemorrhage

IVH (intraventricular haemorrhage) is the most common and serious lesion.

IVH

This is a lesion of the premature infant with an incidence of 40% in infants weighing less than 1500 g or under 32 weeks' gestation. The most common site is the germinal matrix at the junction of the head of the caudate nucleus and choroid plexus in the floor of the lateral ventricle (caudothalamic groove).

The germinal matrix is a highly vascular structure which is present in premature but not term infants. The vessels are prone to injury. Bleeding into the germinal matrix may rupture through the ependyma resulting in intraventricular haemorrhage which may lead to post haemorrhagic hydrocephalus.

Optimal scanning for detection of PVH-IVH is 4–7 days after birth with a follow-up scan at 14 days.

The germinal matrix

Highly vascular structure with thin-walled friable vessels. The vascular supply is sensitive to fluctuations in arterial blood pressures. Ischaemia increases cerebral blood flow leading to distension of fragile arterioles and capillaries. Elevations in venous pressure also predispose the vessels in the germinal matrix to rupture. Elevated venous pressure is usually the result of myocardial failure due to perinatal asphyxia or elevated intrathoracic pressure particularly secondary to pneumothorax.

Hypoxia or ischaemia leads to hyperperfusion or venous distension, followed by increased vascular pressure and then rupture of vessels in the germinal matrix.

CLINICAL PRESENTATION

Diminished consciousness levels.

Hypotonia, seizures, apnoea, coma.

GRADING OF INTRACRANIAL HAEMORRHAGE

Grade 1 – confined to the subependymal matrix.

Grade 2 – intraventricular haemorrhage without ventricular dilatation.

Grade 3 – IVH with ventricular dilatation.

Grade 4 – IVH with intraparenchymal haemorrhage.

ULTRASOUND APPEARANCES
Grade 1
Subependymal haemorrhage.

- Appears echogenic due to formation of fibrin mesh within the organised clot.

- On coronal scans the echogenic focus is observed inferiorly to the floor of the frontal horn (Fig. 2.14a).

- On parasagittal sections the SEH appears as a bulge anterior to the termination of the caudothalamic groove (Fig. 2.14b).

- May be unilateral or bilateral.

Grade 2
- Haemorrhage into a non-dilated ventricle appears as intensely echogenic material within part of, or all of, the ventricular system (Fig. 2.15).

- A small blood clot may settle in the dependent part of the ventricle, i.e. the occipital horn of the lateral ventricle (Fig. 2.16).

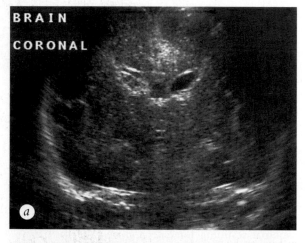

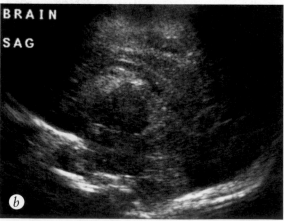

Figure 2.14 — Coronal (a) and right parasagittal (b) sections showing subependymal haemorrhage (Grade I).

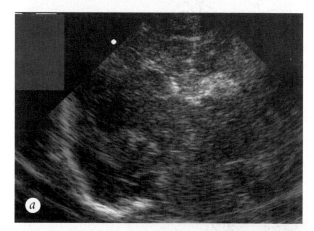

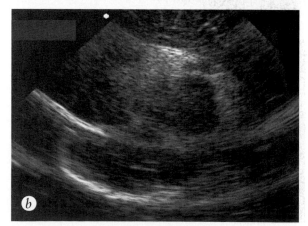

Figure 2.15 — Coronal (a) and left parasagittal (b) sections showing intraventricular haemorrhage within all of the left non-dilated ventricle (Grade II).

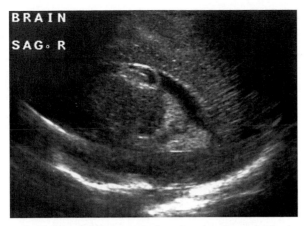

Figure 2.16 — Right parasagittal section showing a clot in the occipital horn of the right lateral ventricle adjacent to the choroid plexus.

- IVH most likely originates in the choroid plexus and although it may occur in premature infants, choroid plexus haemorrhage is more frequent in term infants.

- The diagnosis of isolated choroid plexus haemorrhage may be difficult because the choroid plexus is normally echogenic and bulbous.

- Look for an irregular contour of the choroid plexus, loss of tapering of the anterior caudothalamic groove, and extension of choroid plexus into the occipital horn. Any of these should raise the suspicion of IV clot adherent to choroid.

Grade 3
- Diagnosis of IVH becomes easier as the ventricles dilate (Fig. 2.17).

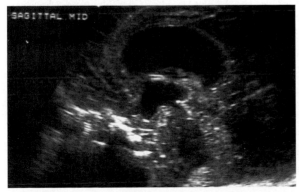

Figure 2.17 — Sagittal section showing haemorrhage within the lateral ventricle leading to post haemorrhagic hydrocephalus (Grade III).

- Blood within dilated ventricles is most often observed within the body extending posteriorly for a variable extent.

- With severe IVH the ventricle is completely filled with echogenic blood and has a cast-like appearance.

- The distended frontal, occipital and temporal horns are readily identifiable on parasagittal sections.

- Coronal images confirm the findings on parasagittal images.

- IVH may be bilateral and symmetrical or it may be confined to one ventricle.

- In severe cases the third and fourth ventricles also fill with blood.

Grade 4
- Intraparenchymal haemorrhage appears as an intensely echogenic focus adjacent to the lateral ventricle, most commonly in the frontal and parietal lobes.

- With large IPH, mass effect, with shift of the midline structures to the unaffected contralateral side, may be observed.

- Haemorrhage as it is resorbed decreases in echogeni-city, fragments and retracts.

- Liquefication occurs 1–2 weeks after a large haemorrhage and appears hypoechoic with an echogenic rim.

PROGNOSIS

Grade	1	2	3	4
Mortality	15%	20%	40%	60%
Incidence of ventricular dilatation	5%	25%	55%	80%
Incidence of long-term neurological sequelae	15%	30%	40%	90%

Intracerebellar haemorrhage

More frequent in premature infants, this is an uncommon but serious lesion.

Possible causes are: ischaemia, traumatic forceps or breech deliveries, direct occipital compression by compressive straps for face mask ventilation.

ULTRASOUND APPEARANCES
- Best identified on coronal scan.

- Loss of definition of the normal posterior fossa landmarks.

- The cerebellum appears asymmetrically echogenic with altered parenchymal echotexture.

Intracerebral haemorrhage

Isolated intracerebral haemorrhage without PVH-IVH occurs in term infants in association with trauma.

It is almost always supratentorial and frequently associated with extraaxial haemorrhage.

ULTRASOUND APPEARANCES
- An abnormal area of increased echogenicity in the cerebral cortex.

Extracerebral fluid collections

Excessive fluid over and between the cerebral hemispheres which is best imaged beneath the anterior fontanelle.

CLINICAL PRESENTATION
Large head.

CHOICE OF TRANSDUCER
10 MHz linear transducer.

ULTRASOUND APPEARANCES
- Fluid collection varies from hypoechoic to echogenic depending upon the nature of the fluid, i.e. CSF or haemorrhage.
- Interhemispheric subdural collections can be seen as fluid between the two hemispheres (Fig. 2.18).
- Subdural blood has a 'V' configuration in the falx under the fontanelle and layers out on the subarachnoid membrane without interdigitation with the sulci.

It is important to differentiate between subdural and subarachnoid fluid/haemorrhage.

- Colour Doppler can be used to differentiate between a subdural and arachnoid collection. Vascular flow can be seen in arachnoid vessels crossing the subarachnoid spaces whilst no vessels cross a subdural space.

Associated findings: flattened gyri, distorted and compressed ventricles.

Subarachnoid

More frequent in term infants than in premature, this is

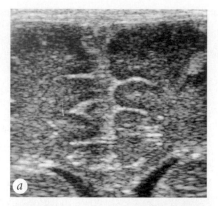

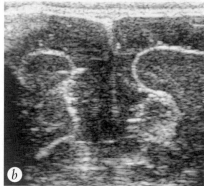

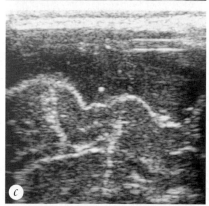

Figure 2.18 — Linear coronal sections showing (a) normal appearances of the interhemispheric fissure and (b) widening of the interhemispheric fissure due to a subdural haemorrhage. (c) Linear sagittal section showing subdural collection.

related to asphyxia or trauma and may be a feature of communicating hydrocephalus. There is variability of the amount of subarachnoid fluid in normal infants. Finding of 'excess' must be related to clinical picture. It can be difficult to demonstrate. Acute subarachnoid blood may be seen to underlie a subdural haemorrhage (Fig. 2.19).

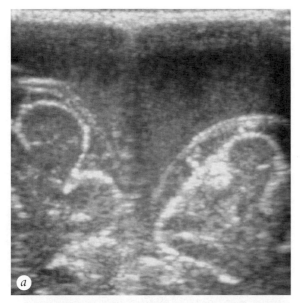

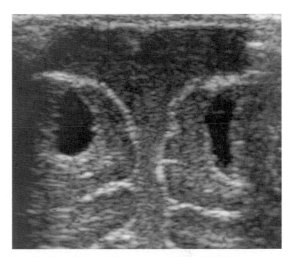

Figure 2.20 — Near field scanning with a 10 MHz transducer demonstrates cystic lesions representing delicate contusional shearing injuries at the corticomedullary junction of the right and left frontal lobe.

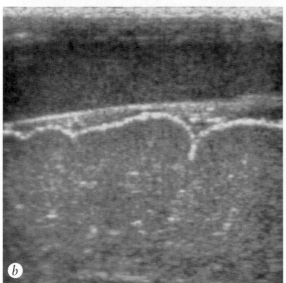

Figure 2.19 — Linear coronal (a) and sagittal (b) sections showing subarachnoid and subdural collections.

PITFALLS

The sagittal sinus should not be mistaken for a subdural collection.

LIMITATIONS

Small haematomas and posterior fossa collections may be difficult to diagnose because of the inability to angle the transducer sufficiently to image the lateral and posterior surfaces of the brain reliably. Ultrasound cannot differentiate between sterile subdural effusion or empyema; although clinically the patient will have a fever if there is empyema. CT/MRI is required.

Hypoxic ischaemic encephalopathy

Decreased oxygen content of the blood and a decrease in cerebral blood flow.

Causes morbidity and death.

CLINICAL PRESENTATION

Asphyxia due to any cause, commonly traumatic delivery, cyanotic heart disease or meconium aspiration.

End result is variable, ranging from normality to cerebral palsy, seizures, mental retardation.

Subdural

This is more frequent in full term infants than in premature. It is related to birth trauma when there is an appropriate history or non-accidental injury (NAI) and is a result of either falx laceration, tearing of bridging veins and tentorial laceration, or a combination of these (Fig. 2.20).

Periventricular leucomalacia (PVL)

This is the primary ischaemic injury in premature infants, as the periventricular white matter is prone to ischaemic damage.

CLINICAL PRESENTATION

Premature infant with history of cerebral ischaemia, cardiorespiratory difficulty, or PVH–IVH.

Cortical visual impairment, spastic diplegia or quadriplegia.

ULTRASOUND APPEARANCES

- Insensitive to subtle changes.
- Increased parenchymal echogenicity adjacent to the frontal horns and trigones of the lateral ventricles (Fig. 2.21).
- Lesions can be unilateral or bilateral and may resolve over a period of 2–3 weeks or may develop into periventricular cysts.
- Cysts appear thick walled and multiple and usually do not communicate with the ventricular system (Fig. 2.22).
- If, however, the ependymal lining breaks down, the cysts can communicate with the lateral ventricles producing ventricular diverticula.
- Late findings include cerebral atrophy, prominence of the cerebral sulci and varying degrees of ventriculomegaly.

PITFALLS

The increased periventricular echogenicity that occurs with PVL must be differentiated from the normal periventricular echogenic halo or blush seen in neonates.

Normal halo–homogeneous, ill-defined borders with an echogenicity less than that of the choroid plexus.

PVL – echogenicity is more intense, heterogeneous and discretely defined.

In some instances a definitive diagnosis may require follow-up scans and a demonstration of periventricular cysts.

Posterior fossa anomalies

Include Dandy-Walker malformation, Dandy-Walker

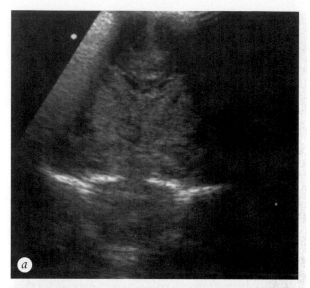

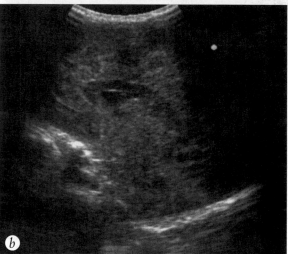

Figure 2.21 — Coronal (a) and sagittal (b) sections showing increased parenchymal echogenicity adjacent to the frontal horns and trigones of lateral ventricles.

variant and the mega-cisterna magna, thought to be caused by insults to the developing cerebellum and 4th ventricle.

CLINICAL PRESENTATION

Increased head circumference.

Hydrocephalus.

Developmental delay.

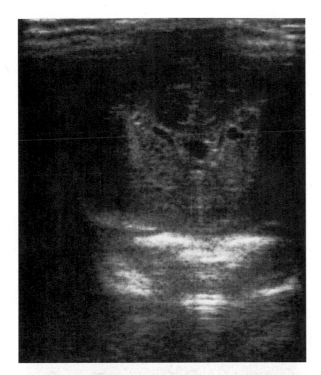

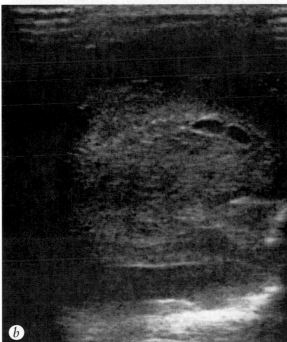

Figure 2.22 — Evolving periventricular leucomalacia: (a) coronal section showing multiple cysts adjacent to the left frontal horn; (b) sagittal section showing small cystic lesions adjacent to the lateral angle of the left ventricle.

Dandy-Walker malformation (Fig. 2.23).

ULTRASOUND APPEARANCES

- Enlarged posterior fossa containing a large fluid-filled anechoic cyst communicating with the 4th ventricle.
- Partial or complete absence of the cerebellar vermis.
- Hypoplasia and anterolateral displacement of the cerebellar hemispheres.
- Elevation of the tentorium.
- Dilatation of the third and lateral ventricles.

Dandy-Walker variant

ULTRASOUND APPEARANCES

- Vermis less hypoplastic.

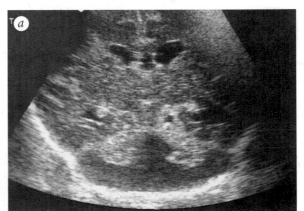

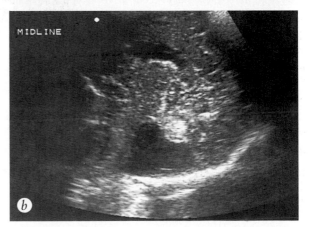

Figure 2.23 — Dandy-Walker malformation. Coronal section (a) showing a large defect where the vermis should be located; (b) midline sagittal section through the posterior fossa showing a small, high cerebellum and cystic fourth ventricle.

- Normal sized posterior fossa.
- Cystic dilatation of the fourth ventricle.

Mega-cisterna magna

ULTRASOUND APPEARANCES

- Intact vermis.
- Enlarged posterior fossa secondary to an enlarged cisterna magna.
- No dilatation of fourth ventricle.

PITFALLS

Dandy-Walker malformation must be distinguished from a posterior fossa arachnoid cyst.

An arachnoid cyst will show an intact cerebellar vermis and no communication with the fourth ventricle.

ASSOCIATED ANOMALIES

Congenital cardiac abnormalities.

Polydactyly.

Encephalocele

An encephalocele is a dysraphic disorder and is herniation of intracranial contents through a defect in the skull. Most are located midline occurring in the occipital region but can also occur in parietal, nasal and frontal regions.

ULTRASOUND APPEARANCES

- Typically rounded anechoic or complex mass depending on the extent of herniated soft tissue.

MERITS

Although encephalocele can be diagnosed clinically, ultrasound is useful in determining the amount of brain tissue contained within the sac preoperatively. CT/MRI may also be useful.

ASSOCIATED ABNORMALITIES

Encephalocele may be an isolated anomaly.

May be associated with Dandy-Walker malformation, diastematomyelia or Klippel-Feil syndrome.

Vein of Galen malformation

This is an arteriovenous malformation caused by the failure of embryonic arteriovenous shunts to be replaced by capillaries. Increased blood flow is therefore shunted directly from the arteries into the deep venous system.

CLINICAL PRESENTATION

Cardiac failure.

Hydrocephalus.

Seizures/headaches.

ULTRASOUND APPEARANCES

- Well circumscribed anechoic mass in the midline, posterior to the third ventricle and superior to the vermis (Fig. 2.24 a, b).
- Colour flow Doppler studies can confirm the increased flow in the vein of Galen (Fig. 2.24c).
- CT or MRI is required to confirm diagnosis with angiography to define the full extent of the malformation and to plan treatment.

PITFALLS

The dilated vein could be confused with an arachnoid cyst, therefore colour Doppler is essential to differentiate.

TREATMENT

Embolisation and subsequent surgery.

Brain tumours

Though occasionally identified by ultrasound as a hyperechoic mass lesion, relatively few occur prior to fontanelle closure and are therefore not identified often by ultrasound.

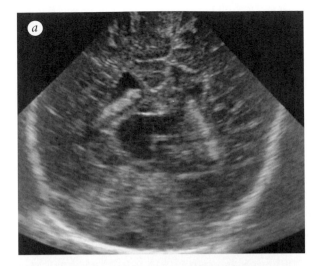

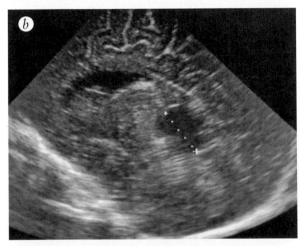

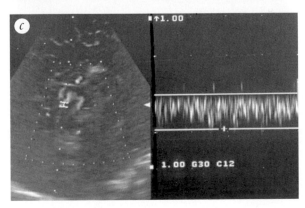

Figure 2.24 — Coronal (a) and lateral (b) views showing a well-circumscribed anechoic mass in the midline, posterior to the third ventricle and superior to the vermis. (c) Colour flow Doppler confirms the dilated vein of Galen.

Further reading

Bowerman RA, Zwischenberger JB, Andrews AF, Bartlett RH. Cranial sonography of the infant treated with extracorporeal membrane oxygenation. *AJR* 1985; **145**: 161–166.

Bowerman RA, Donn SM, DiPietro MA, D'DAmato CJ, Hicks SP. Periventricular leukomalacia in the pre-term newborn infant: sonographic and clinical features. *Radiology* 1984; **151**: 383–388.

Bowie JD, Kirks DR, Rosenberg ER, Clair MR. Caudothalamic groove: value in identification of germinal matrix hemorrhage by sonography in preterm neonates. *AJR* 1983; **141**: 1317–1320.

Chambers SE, Hendry GM, Wild SR. Real time ultrasound scanning of the head in neonates and infants, including a correlation between ultrasound and computed tomography. *Pediatr Radiol* 1985; **15**(1): 4–7.

Chen C, Chou T, Zimmerman RA, Lee C, Chen F, Faro SH. Pericerebral fluid collections: differentiation of enlarged subarachnoid spaces from subdural collections with colour doppler US. *Radiology* 1996; **201**: 389–392.

Cohen MD, Slabaugh RD, Smith JA, Jansen R, Greenman GF, Macdonald N, Reider JI. Neurosonographic identification of ventricular asymmetry in premature infants. *Clin Radiol* 1984; **35**(1): 29–31.

D'Souza SW, Gowland M, Richards B, Cadman J, Mellor V, Sims DG, Chiswick ML. Head size, brain growth, and lateral ventricles in very low birthweight infants. *Arch Dis Child* 1986; **61**(11): 1090–1095.

Goodwin L, Quisling RG. The neonatal cisterna magna: ultrasonic evaluation. *Radiology* 1983; **149**(3): 691–695.

Gray's Anatomy: the anatomical basis of medicine and surgery. 38th ed. Edinburgh: Churchill Livingstone, 1995.

Jaspan T, Narborough G, Punt JAG et al. Cerebral contusional tears as a marker of child abuse – detection by cranial sonography. *Pediatr Radiol* 1992; **22**: 237–245.

Jaspan T. Cranial ultrasound in non-accidental injury. *BMUS Bulletin* 1998; **6**(3): 29–38.

Levene MI, Starte DR. A longitudinal study of post-haemorrhagic ventricular dilatation in the newborn. *Arch Dis Child* 1981; **56**(12): 905–910.

Libicher M, Troger J. US measurement of the subarachnoid space in infants: normal values. *Radiology* 1992; **184**: 749–751.

Mack LA, Rumack CM, Johnson ML. Ultrasound evaluation of cystic intracranial lesions in the neonate. *Radiology* 1980; **137**(2): 451–455.

McLeary RD, Kuhns LR, Barr M Jr. Ultrasonography of the fetal cerebellum. *Radiology* 1984; **151**(2): 439–442.

Nyberg DA, Cyr DR, Mack LA, Fitzsimmons J, Hickok D, Mahony BS. The Dandy-Walker malformation: prenatal sonographic diagnosis and its clinical significance. *J Ultrasound Med* 1988; **7**(2): 65–71.

O'Donnabhain D, Duff DF. Aneurysms of the vein of Galen. *Arch Dis Child* 1989; **64**(11): 1612–1617.

Rumack CM, Horgan JG, Hay TC, Kindsfater D. *Pocket Atlas of Pediatric Ultrasound*. New York, Raven Press, 1990.

Rumack CM, Manco-Johnson ML, Manco-Johnson MJ, Koops BL, Hathaway WE, Appareti K. Timing and course of neonatal intracranial hemorrhage using real-time ultrasound. *Radiology* 1985; **154**: 101–105.

Saliba E, Bertrand P, Gold F, Marchand S, Laugier J. Area of lateral ventricles measured on cranial ultrasonography in preterm infants: association with outcome. *Arch Dis Child* 1990; **65**: 1033–1037.

Saunders AJS. Cranial ultrasound in infants. *BMUS Bulletin* 1998; **6**(3): 17–27.

Siegel M. *Pediatric Sonography*. New York, 2nd ed. Raven Press, 1995.

Siegel MJ, Shackelford GD, Perlman JM, Fulling KH. Hypoxic-ischemic encephalopathy in term infants: diagnosis and prognosis evaluated by ultrasound. *Radiology* 1984; **152**: 395–399.

Szymonowicz W, Yu VY. Timing and evolution of periventricular haemorrhage in infants weighing 1250 g or less at birth. *Arch Dis Child* 1984; **59**(1): 7–12.

Taylor GA, Madsen JR. Neonatal hydrocephalus: hemodynamic response to fontanelle compression – correlation with intracranial pressure and need for shunt placement. *Radiology* 1996; **201**: 685–689.

Wilson ME, Lindsay DJ, Levi CS, Ackerman TE, Gordon WL. US case of the day. Dandy-Walker variant with agenesis of the corpus callosum. *Radiographics* 1994; **14**(3): 678–681.

3

THE
NECK AND FACE

SALIVARY GLANDS

Anatomy

There are three major groups : submandibular, parotid and sublingual.

Submandibular

This is bordered by the mandible laterally and the mylohyoid muscle superiorly and medially. Drained by duct of Wharton.

Parotid

The largest gland is superficial and lies between the ramus of the mandible anteriorly and the mastoid process and sternocleidomastoid muscle pos-teriorly. Subdivided into lateral (80% of gland) and medial (20%) lobe separated by the facial nerve.

Drained by duct of Stennsen which runs along anterior border of the gland; it crosses the masseter muscle to enter the oral cavity.

Sublingual

These lie deep in the mylohyoid muscle and are multiple.

CHOICE OF TRANSDUCER
10 MHz linear.

PATIENT PREPARATION
None.

ULTRASOUND APPEARANCES OF NORMAL SALIVARY GLANDS
- *Submandibular* – Similar in echotexture to the normal parotid. It is more hyperechoic than a lymph node (Fig. 3.1).
- *Parotid* – Elliptical shape: more homogeneous and hyperechoic than adjacent muscle due to fatty glandular tissue. Facial artery can be seen in the superficial portion (Fig. 3.2).
- *Sublingual* – Not usually identified unless enlarged.

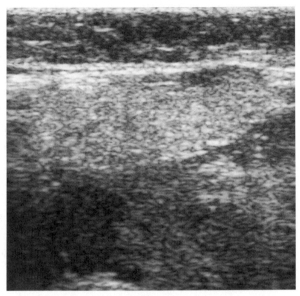

Figure 3.1 — Normal submandibular gland. The texture of the normal parotid gland is similar.

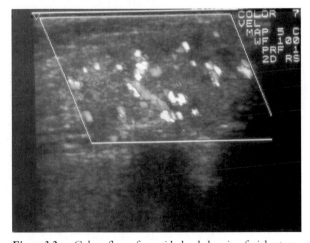

Figure 3.2 — Colour flow of parotid gland showing facial artery.

CLINICAL PROBLEMS

Sialectasis

ULTRASOUND APPEARANCES
- The gland is enlarged.
- There are multiple small hypoechoic lesions due to dilated acini (Fig. 3.3).
- Stones may occur in these and cast acoustic shadows.
- Small lymph nodes within the glands are often seen.

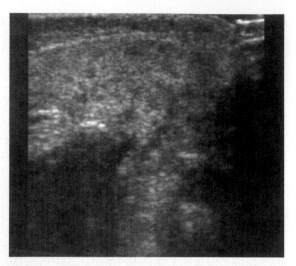

Figure 3.3 — Sialectasis of the parotid gland. The small hypoechoic areas are dilated acini.

Tumour

Parotid gland tumours are rare in children.

ULTRASOUND APPEARANCES

- They are solid and are seen as areas of altered echogenicity compared with normal tissue.
- The neck should be examined for lymph nodes.
- Reactive enlargement may occur with chemotherapy.

Haemangioma of the parotid gland

This is a benign vascular tumour within the gland.

ULTRASOUND APPEARANCES

- Calcific opacities are frequent.
- The lesion usually infiltrates the tissue without clear margin.
- Colour flow mapping should be done.

Ranula

A submandibular mass due to blockage of a sublingual duct in the floor of the mouth with the accumulated secretions forming the mass.

ULTRASOUND APPEARANCES

There is a smooth avascular hypoechoic but not fluid-filled mass lying close to the submandibular gland (Fig. 3.4).

THYROID GLAND

Anatomy

There are two lateral lobes, one either side of the trachea, connected by isthmus anterior to the trachea.

The size varies with age. In transverse section it measures 1–1.5 cm. The right lobe is usually larger than the left.

PATIENT PREPARATION

None.

TECHNIQUE

The patient is supine with chin hyperextended and shoulders raised on pillows to help extend the neck. The transducer is placed over the anterior mid neck in transverse section and movements are made until the thyroid gland is located. The transducer should be angled cranio-caudally to image the entire gland. The transducer is rotated 90 degrees and each lobe is imaged in longitudinal section.

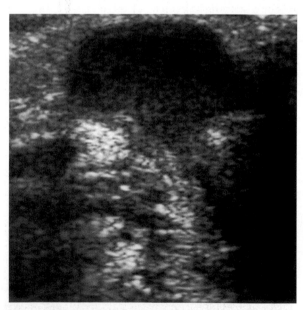

Figure 3.4 — Ranula. Typical appearance of a cystic mass with some internal echoes, lying under the mandible, lateral to the submandibular gland (not shown).

Measurements of the lobes in longitudinal and transverse sections should be made.

ULTRASOUND APPEARANCES

- The gland appears as a homogeneous, two-lobed structure with a connecting isthmus (Fig. 3.5).

- It is hyperechoic compared to neck muscles.

- It is bordered posterolaterally by the CCA (common carotid artery) and the IJV (internal jugular vein), medially by the trachea and oesophagus and antero-laterally by the sternocleidomastoid muscle (Fig. 3.6).

MERITS

Ultrasound can demonstrate the presence or absence of the gland, distinguish between solitary or multiple nodules and between solid nodules and cysts. It identifies an enlarged gland and shows any abnormal echogenicity which indicates inflammation or thyroiditis.

Goitre

A goitre is an enlarged thyroid gland.

CLINICAL PRESENTATION

Diffuse swelling is present in the anterior neck. The patient may be euthyroid, hypothyroid or hyperthyroid.

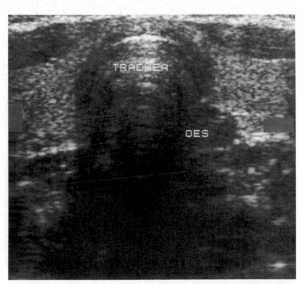

Figure 3.5 — Transverse section of a normal thyroid. Midline section (oes = oesophagus). The right and left lobes are shown.

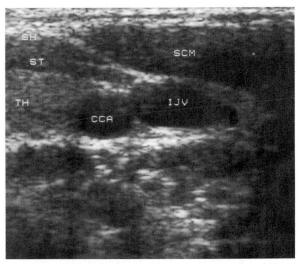

Figure 3.6 — Transverse section lateral part of left lobe.

CCA = Common carotid artery   SH = Sternohyoid muscle
IJV = Internal jugular vein   ST = Sternothyroid
SCM = Sternocleidomastoid muscle

TECHNIQUE

As for normal thyroid.

ULTRASOUND APPEARANCES

Simple goitre

- Diffusely enlarged with normal echo-texture.

- Colour flow imaging can be useful to demonstrate any hypervascularity of the gland and its extent (Fig. 3.7).

- Hypervascularity is seen in a hyperactive gland and in inflammatory situations.

Multinodular goitre

This is due to repeated hyperplasia and involution

- The gland is heterogeneous with both echogenic and cystic areas.

This condition is rare in children.

Cyst

Simple cyst

A simple cyst is rare in children and represents about 1% of benign thyroid masses.

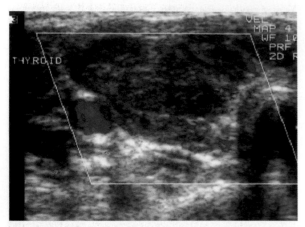

Figure 3.7 — Simple goitre. Diffusely enlarged right lobe of thyroid. Note hypervascularity.

Most cysts are the result of degeneration of a follicular adenoma.

CLINICAL PRESENTATION

There is a palpable smooth neck mass which moves with swallowing.

TECHNIQUE

As for normal thyroid gland.

ULTRASOUND APPEARANCES
- Hypoechoic/sonolucent mass with smooth walls.
- Post-cystic enhancement is present due to through transmission of ultrasound.
- It is avascular on colour flow.

TREATMENT

Usually aspiration under ultrasound control, with subsequent monitoring to exclude recurrence.

Haemorrhagic cyst

Acute haemorrhage into follicular adenoma. It may be due to trauma but more usually develops spontaneously.

ULTRASOUND APPEARANCES
- There is a hyperechoic, complex mass which may contain internal septae and debris.
- The walls are initially irregular but become more circumscribed.
- A fluid level is sometimes found.

Adenoma

This is the most common benign neoplasm and is due to hyperplasia and involution of a thyroid lobule.

ULTRASOUND APPEARANCES
- The nodule is hypoechoic (some may be hyperechoic or isoechoic).
- 60% demonstrate a thin (1–2 mm) sonolucent rim around the lesion.
- It may contain small cystic areas due to haemorrhage and necrosis (Fig. 3.8).
- Calcification, though rare, appears in the periphery as bright echogenic foci with associated acoustic shadowing.
- Colour flow imaging demonstrates a vascular rim.

Thyroiditis

Bacterial thyroiditis

This is rare in children and is associated with a congenital pyriform sinus fistula which becomes infected. Age range 2–12 years.

CLINICAL PRESENTATION

Enlarged, tender gland, often affecting the left lobe.

ULTRASOUND APPEARANCES
- A hypoechoic mass, which may be single or multiple with an enlarged thyroid lobe.

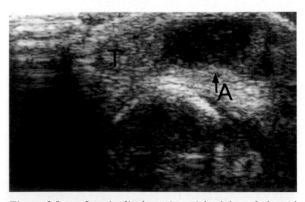

Figure 3.8 — Longitudinal section right lobe of thyroid containing hypoechoic central adenoma. T = thyroid lobe. A = adenoma.

Hashimoto's (lymphocytic) thyroiditis

An organ specific autoimmune disease affecting adolescent girls and women older than 40 years.

CLINICAL PRESENTATION

Painless enlargement of the thyroid gland. Most affected children are euthyroid at presentation with normal thyroid function tests, but ultimately become hypothyroid.

ULTRASOUND APPEARANCES

- The gland is enlarged, with a multinodular mixed echoic appearance, the nodules being hypoechoic (Fig. 3.9).
- Colour flow shows hypervascularity (Fig. 3.10).
- Lymphadenopathy may be present in the adjoining lymph nodes.

Thyroglossal cyst

This is a remnant of a track left behind during development of the thyroid from the branchial arch. Clinically, the cyst is midline and moves with the thyroid gland (Fig. 3.11). It may become infected and an abscess may develop.

ULTRASOUND APPEARANCES

- A small midline cystic structure is present, which moves with the thyroid gland.
- A track between the cyst and the thyroid gland may be identified.

TREATMENT
Surgical excision is required.

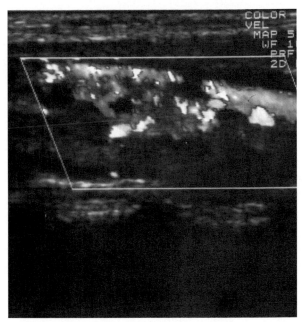

Figure 3.10 — Hashimoto's thyroiditis. Colour flow shows hypervascularity of gland.

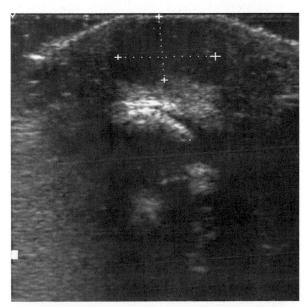

Figure 3.11 — Midline thyroglossal cyst lying in the isthmus.

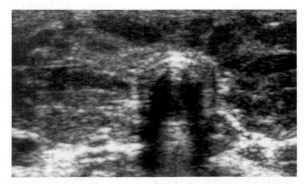

Figure 3.9 — Hashimoto's thyroiditis, transverse section. Note diffusely enlarged gland and isthmus with multiple hypoechoic though not cystic areas. Note absence of normal tissue.

INFLAMMATORY SWELLING IN THE NECK

Lymphadenitis

Inflammatory enlarged lymph nodes as a result of infection from the nearby pharyngeal structures, e.g. tonsils or dental pathology. The child presents with a firm painful mass.

CHOICE OF TRANSDUCER

10 MHz linear array.

ULTRASOUND APPEARANCES

- Hypoechoic round or oval masses greater than 5 mm in diameter (Fig. 3.12).
- The hilum of the lymph gland can be seen as an echogenic line in the centre of the lymph node (Fig. 3.13).
- Colour flow imaging is useful to differentiate between small nodes and vessels.
- The nodes are avascular except for colour flow from the central hilar vessel.
- If they contain calcification, tuberculosis should be suggested.

TREATMENT

Antibiotics.

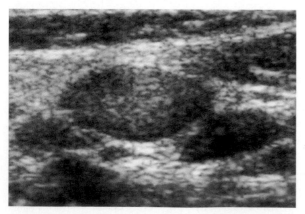

Figure 3.12 — Multiple discrete normal lymph nodes in the neck.

Abscess

This results from suppuration of an infected lymph node.

ULTRASOUND APPEARANCES

- There is a well-defined, thick-walled, partial or totally fluid-filled mass (Fig. 3.14a, b).
- Gas bubbles which may be present appear echogenic with shadowing in the abscess centre.
- Colour flow imaging demonstrates flow around the periphery with no flow in the centre.

TREATMENT

Surgical drainage and antibiotics. Percutaneous aspiration can be undertaken under ultrasound control to obtain material for microbiology.

Calcification does not occur in simple infective lymph nodes but may be seen in healing tuberculous nodes.

LIMITATIONS

The source of infection, e.g. sinuses or retropharynx, cannot be demonstrated with ultrasound.

Malignant lymphadenopathy

Lymphoma is the most frequent cause of malignant lymphadenopathy in the neck. Other causes include

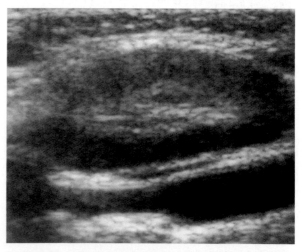

Figure 3.13 — Longitudinal section of a normal node with an echogenic hilum.

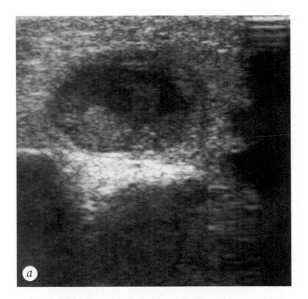

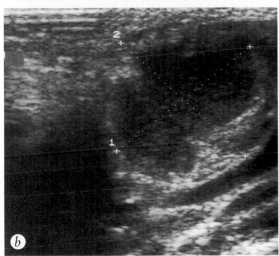

Figure 3.14 — Abscess in (a) the pre-auricular region and (b) the neck. Note the irregular thick walled masses containing fluid with internal echoes due to the pus. In (b) the mass lies in front of the neck vessels.

metastatic spread from nasopharyngeal and retropharyngeal rhabdomyosarcoma and primitive neuro-ectodermal tumours (PNETs). Rarely an abdominal neuroblastoma may present with supraclavicular nodes. A high paravertebral neuroblastoma may have direct extension into the neck.

CLINICAL PRESENTATION
Palpable neck mass.

ULTRASOUND APPEARANCES
- Enlarged lymph nodes greater than 5 mm in diameter with a homogeneous or heterogeneous texture.

- The nodes are often not discrete; if so, this helps to distinguish benign from malignant disease.

TREATMENT
Biopsy to confirm diagnosis.

LIMITATIONS
CT or MR must be performed to determine the location and extent of the disease for full staging.

If lymphoma is suspected on ultrasound examination, the abdomen should be examined to assess splenic or renal involvement.

CONGENITAL AND DEVELOPMENTAL ABNORMALITIES

Cystic hygroma

A congenital malformation of primitive lymphatic channels of unknown aetiology. The neck is a frequent site. Pathologically, there are large cysts of varying sizes lined with a single layer of endothelium: 75% are found in the neck and 20% in the axilla, with the remainder in the mediastinum, retroperitoneum and abdominal viscera. Many lesions are mixed haemangiomas/lymphangiomas and have a propensity to haemorrhage into the cyst and therefore fluctuate in size and echotexture.

CHOICE OF TRANSDUCER:
10 MHz linear array.

CLINICAL PRESENTATION
They commonly present at or shortly after birth as a painless, soft tissue mass posterior to the SCM. It may fill one side of the neck and extend into the mediastinum producing oesophageal or airway compression.

ULTRASOUND APPEARANCES
- An uncomplicated lesion appears as a thin-walled mass which may be a solitary cyst or contain multiple cysts with septa of variable thickness (Fig. 3.15).

- It may contain echogenic fluid if recent haemorrhage has occurred.

- The margins may be poorly defined if the lesion infiltrates the adjacent structures.

- Colour flow imaging demonstrates an avascular mass and defines the relationship to the nearby major vessels (Fig. 3.15).

- A mixed lesion with haemangioma will have mixed solid and cystic components (Fig. 3.16).

TREATMENT
Surgical drainage.

MERITS
The ultrasonic appearance is diagnostic but it should be supplemented with MR to identify the full extent, especially mediastinal extension. Ultrasonic monitoring will show the presence of recent haemorrhage or infection, this explaining the size alteration.

These cysts may be aspirated under ultrasound control, providing therapeutic relief.

Haemangioma

This is a developmental vascular abnormality occurring anywhere on the body. It is found in infants younger than 6 months of age but is not present at birth. It

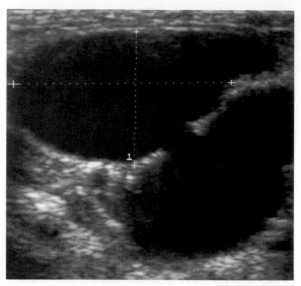

Figure 3.16 — Typical appearance of complex cystic hygroma. Note septae. The fluid is transonic indicating that there has been no haemorrhage.

frequently regresses spontaneously in childhood. There are two types:

Capillary with capillary sized vascular spaces with few erythrocytes.

Cavernous with larger dilated erythrocyte filled vascular spaces but without major feeding vessels.

Both types may be localised to the skin or involve the deeper soft tissues of the neck.

CLINICAL PRESENTATION
Strawberry 'birthmark'. This is slightly misleading as the lesion is not present at birth but may develop in the first few days. There is a blue tinge to the skin, with an ill defined mass.

ULTRASOUND APPEARANCES

Capillary haemangiomas

Echogenic due to numerous interfaces, proteinaceous material or areas of thrombosis and fibrosis. Colour flow imaging demonstrates minimal, if any, blood flow.

Cavernous haemangiomas (Fig. 3.17a)

Complex masses with anechoic areas separated by echogenic tissue. They may be well defined or infiltrate

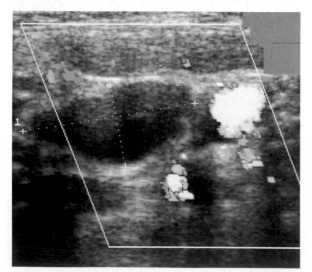

Figure 3.15 — Single cyst cystic hygroma lying medial to the carotid artery.

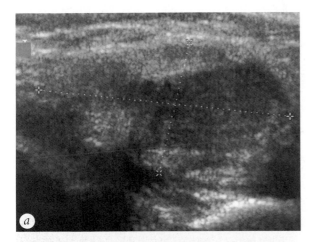

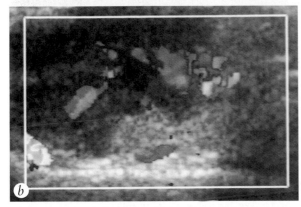

Figure 3.17 — (a) Cavernous haemangioma in neck, seen as irregular hypoechoic mass, with some echogenic areas and poorly defined borders, where it infiltrates surrounding tissues. (b) Colour flow through the lesion shows feeding vessels.

normal structures. Colour flow imaging may demonstrate feeding arteries but not always. (Fig. 3.17b).

Branchial cyst

This is an embryological remnant of a branchial arch malformation and presents as a palpable cystic mass in the neck, lateral to the midline. It may have an associated sinus and become infected. The reason for ultrasound is to distinguish this from a thyroglossal cyst. A branchial cyst will always be separate from the thyroid.

CHOICE OF TRANSDUCER
10 MHz linear array.

ULTRASOUND APPEARANCES
- If not infected, a well defined transonic smooth walled cyst (Fig. 3.18) is seen separate from the thyroid gland.
- If infected, it then has a heterogeneous appearance like any abscess.

TREATMENT
Surgical excision is required.

Fibromatosis colli

CLINICAL PRESENTATION
Congenital contraction and infiltration of the sternomastoid muscle by fibromatous tissue leading to a congenital torticollis concave to the affected side.

TECHNIQUE
The sternomastoid is examined in longitudinal and transverse planes and the extent of the mass measured. Ideally a 10 MHz linear array transducer should be used but if it is too big then a phased array or curvilinear is a better choice.

ULTRASOUND APPEARANCES
- The sternomastoid is shortened and contracted.
- The normal muscle fibres are absent and replaced by an amorphous mass of increased echogenicity with normal muscle above and below it (Fig. 3.19).

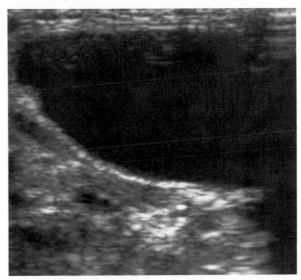

Figure 3.18 — Branchial cyst. Smooth wall anechoic lesion as this is not infected.

- It is technically difficult to demonstrate normal muscle tissue above and below due to tight neck position.

TREATMENT

Initially, physiotherapy but may need surgical division.

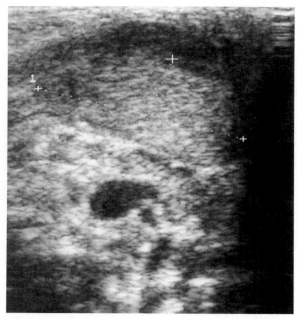

Figure 3.19 — Fibromatosis colli. Note the echogenic lesion within the sternomastoid muscle.

Further reading

Chan YL, Cheng JCY, Metreweli C. Ultrasonography of congenital muscular torticollis. *Pediatr Radiol* 1992; **22**: 356–360.

Cox MR, Marshall SG, Spence RA. Solitary thyroid nodule: a prospective evaluation of nuclear scanning and ultrasonography. *Br J Surg* 1991 Jan; **78**(1): 90–3.

Friedman AP, Haller JO, Goodman JD, Nagar H. Sonographic evaluation of non-inflammatory neck masses in children. *Radiology* 1983; **147**: 693–697.

Glasier CM, Seibert JJ, Williamson SL, Seibert RW et al. High resolution ultrasound characterization of soft tissue masses in children. *Pediatr Radiol* 1987; **17**: 233–237.

Kraus R, Han BK, Babcock DS, Oestreich AE. Sonography of neck masses in children. *AJR* 1986; **146**: 609–613.

Latifi HR, Siegel MJ. Colour Doppler flow imaging of pediatric soft tissue masses. *J Ultrasound Med* 1994; **13**: 165–169.

McIvor NP, Freeman JL, Salem S, Elden L, Noyek AM, Bedard YC. Ultrasonography and ultrasound-guided fine-needle aspiration biopsy of head and neck lesions: a surgical perspective. *Laryngoscope* 1994 Jun; **104**(6 Pt.1): 669–674.

Reynolds JH, Wolinski AP. Sonographic appearance of branchial cysts. *Clin Radiol* 1993 Aug; **48**(2): 109–110.

Siegel MJ, Glazer HS, St. Amour TE, Rosenthal DD. Lymphangiomas in children: MR imaging. *Radiology* 1989; **170**: 467–470.

Soberman N, Leonidas JC, Berdon WE et al. Parotid enlargement in children seropositive for human immunodeficiency virus: imaging findings. *AJR* 1991; **157**: 553–556.

Solbiati L, Cioffi V, Ballarati E. Ultrasonography of the neck. *Radiol Clin North Am* 1992; **30**: 941–954.

Vitti P, Rago T, Mazzeo S et al. Thyroid blood flow evaluation by color-flow Doppler sonography distinguishes Graves' disease from Hashimoto's thyroiditis. *J Endocrinol Invest* 1995 Dec; **18**(11): 857–861.

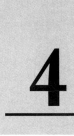

4

THE EYE

PREPARATION

None required.

TRANSDUCER

High frequency 10–7.5 MHz transducer.

High frequency linear transducer may also be useful.

TECHNIQUE

Patient supine. Sterile coupling gel. The transducer is placed gently on the closed eyelid. Both eyes are assessed in sequential sagittal and axial sections, ideally with the globe static and during voluntary movement. A stand-off may be required to image the anterior chamber. Colour doppler will allow assessment of occular and orbital blood flow.

Normal anatomy and ultrasound appearances of the eye (Fig. 4.1a, b)

Anterior chamber: extends from the cornea to the iris and contains aqueous humour which is anechoic.

Posterior chamber: extends from the iris to the posterior surface of the lens. It contains aqueous humour which is anechoic. The lens is anechoic, its posterior and anterior wall are echogenic.

Vitreous chamber: extends from the posterior surface of the lens to the ocular wall, which consists of retina, choroid and sclera. These are echogenic and the different layers cannot be distinguished in the normal eye.

The hypoechoic optic nerve lies at the posterior aspect of the globe within the retrolobar fat, which is echogenic.

Cataract

Partial or complete opacification of the lens of the eye. May be congenital or acquired, e.g. tumour.

CLINICAL PRESENTATION

Opaque lens.

Loss of visual acuity.

ULTRASOUND APPEARANCES (Fig. 4.2)

● Completely echogenic lens.

● A thick rim of increased echogenicity.

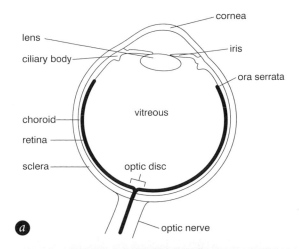

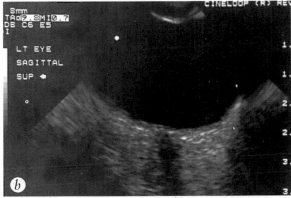

Figure 4.1 — (a) Normal anatomy of the eye. (b) Normal ultrasound appearances of the eye.

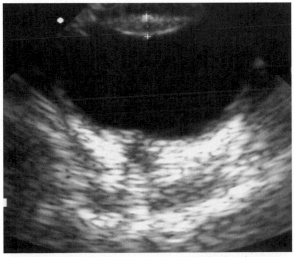

Figure 4.2 — Cataract. The lens appears completely echogenic.

If a plastic lens is implanted following cataract extraction, the eye can still be assessed using ultrasound as long as the implant is avoided.

Retinal detachment

Rare in children and usually traumatic.

Accumulation of fluid between the two layers of the retina. The retinal membrane is fixed at the ora serrata and optic nerve. Detachment does not extend beyond these sites.

CLINICAL PRESENTATION

Trauma.

Diabetes.

Inflammation.

Tumour.

ULTRASOUND APPEARANCES
- Total detachment results in an echogenic V-shaped appearance within the vitreous (Fig. 4.3a).
- Real-time scanning may demonstrate movement.
- Colour flow imaging demonstrates blood flow in the membrane.

Chronic detachment

Fibrosis occurs, the retina becomes immobile and forms a taut membrane between the optic disc and ora serrata (Fig. 4.3b).

Choroidal detachment

Rare in children.

Accumulation of fluid between choroid and sclera in the supra choroidal space.

The choroidal membrane is fixed at the point of exit of the vortex vessels and nerves and anteriorly just beyond the ora serrata.

CLINICAL PRESENTATION

Infection.

Secondary to tumour.

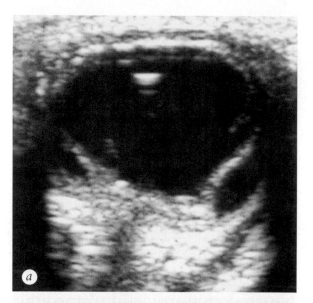

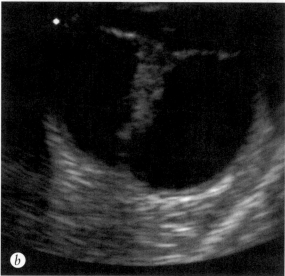

Figure 4.3 — Retinal detachment. (a) The V-shape of the retina is demonstrated following detachment. (b) In chronic detachment the retina is seen as a taut immobile membrane.

ULTRASOUND APPEARANCES
- Convex echogenic membrane within the vitreous.
- Demonstrates blood flow in the membrane.

Posterior vitreous detachment

The gelatinous structure within the vitreous chamber shrinks and separates from the retina. The space created often crosses the optic disc which helps to distinguish it from retinal or choroidal detachment.

CLINICAL PRESENTATION

? Trauma.

Blunt injury.

ULTRASOUND APPEARANCES (Fig. 4.4)

- Real-time ultrasound demonstrates a mobile and deformable vitreous with eye movement.

- Funnel-shaped echogenic structure.

- No colour flow, as the hyaloid is not vascular.

Drusen

Calcified hyaline deposits within the substance of the optic nerve head.

May be congenital or acquired.

Often bilateral.

CLINICAL PRESENTATION

Rarely symptomatic, often discovered incidentally.

Pale, slightly swollen disc at fundoscopy can mimic 'papilloedema'.

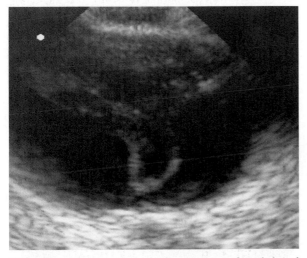

Figure 4.4 — Posterior vitreous detachment. A funnel-shaped echogenic structure within the posterior segment, which on real-time scanning was highly mobile.

ULTRASOUND APPEARANCES (Fig. 4.5)

- Echogenic focus at the optic nerve head.

Persistent hyperplastic primary vitreous (PHPV)

Failure of the embryonic hyaloid vasculature to regress.

Usually unilateral.

ASSOCIATED ANOMALIES

Trisomy 13

Warburg's syndrome

Norrie's disease.

CLINICAL PRESENTATION

Leukaemia.

Microphthalmia.

Small cornea and prominent ciliary processes.

ULTRASOUND APPEARANCES (Fig. 4.6)

- Mild: Echogenic band extending from the posterior surface of the lens to the optic disc.

- Severe: Echogenic mass within the vitreous chamber.

- Highly vascular: Colour doppler demonstrates blood flow within the lesion.

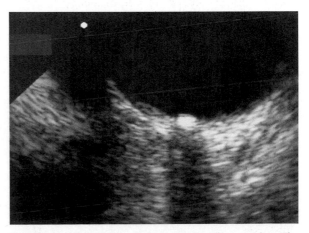

Figure 4.5 — Drusen. An echogenic focus at the optic disc. The hypoechoic optic nerve is seen posteriorly.

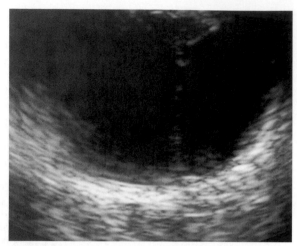

Figure 4.6 — Persistent hyperplastic primary vitreous, an echogenic band extending from the posterior surface of the lens to the optic disc.

- No calcification.
- May be associated with retinal detachment.

Retinoblastoma (Fig. 4.7)

A type of malignant PNET (primitive neuroectodermal tumour) of the retina.

Commonest primary intraocular tumour of childhood.

Average age at presentation 1–2 years but may be congenital.

May be bilateral.

CLINICAL PRESENTATION

- Opaque ocular media.
- Leukocoria (white pupil).

ULTRASOUND APPEARANCES

- Irregular heterogeneous mass involving the retina which projects into the vitreous chamber.
- Calcification.
- May involve the optic nerve.
- May have associated retinal detachment.
- Colour flow and Doppler imaging should be performed to assess blood flow within the lesion.

CT is the imaging modality of choice at initial presentation. However, if intracranial extension is suspected, MRI is indicated. Ultrasound is useful to assess size in serial follow-up.

Trauma

Ultrasound is useful when injury is confined to the globe/soft tissues. CT is the imaging modality of choice when bony injury is suspected.

Ultrasound can help to determine:

- Presence and extent of haemorrhage (see vitreous haemorrhage).
- The location and appearance of the lens (Fig. 4.8).
- Detachment of the retina.
- Presence of a foreign body.

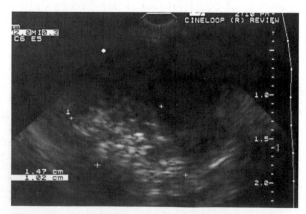

Figure 4.7 — Retinoblastoma, A lobulated echogenic mass arising from the posterior aspect of the globe.

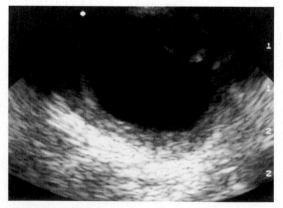

Figure 4.8 — Trauma to the globe demonstrating posterior dislocation of the lens.

A foreign body appears echogenic and causes reverberation artefact.

Vitreous haemorrhage

Bleeding into the vitreous.

CLINICAL PRESENTATION

Opaque media.

Trauma.

Non-accidental injury (Shaken baby syndrome).

Diabetes.

ULTRASOUND APPEARANCES (Fig.4.9)
- Large haemorrhages appear as irregular hyperechoic areas within the anechoic vitreous.
- Small haemorrhages may be difficult to demonstrate.
- May develop fibrinous strands.
- Associated with posterior vitreous detachment.

Inflammatory disorders of the eye

Includes: uveitis, inflammation of the choroid and iris, which is very rare in children.

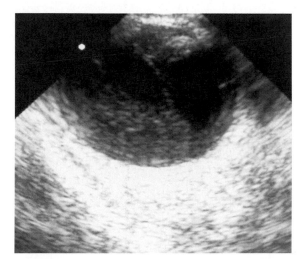

Figure 4.9 — Vitreous haemorrhage. Echogenic debris and fibrinous strands are seen within the vitreous.

CAUSES

Infection – bacterial, viral, TB.

Trauma.

Allergic reaction.

CLINICAL PRESENTATION

Sudden onset of pain.

Redness.

Photophobia of one or both eyes.

ULTRASOUND APPEARANCES (Fig. 4.10)
- May appear normal.
- Low-level echoes within the vitreous.

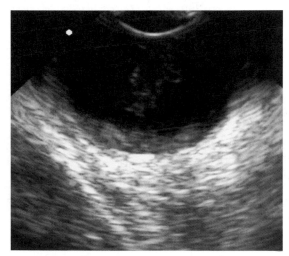

Figure 4.10 — Inflammation. Note the low-level echoes within the vitreous, consistent with inflammatory reaction.

Further reading

Enriquez G, Gil-Gibernau JJ, Garriga V, Ribes I, Lucaya J. Sonography of the eye in children: Imaging findings. *AJR* 1995; **165**: 935–939.

Erickson SJ, Hendrix LE, Massaro BM, Harris GJ, Lewandowski MF, Foley WD, Lawson TL. Color Doppler flow imaging of the normal and abnormal orbit. *Radiology* 1989; **173**: 511–516.

Fielding JA. Pictorial review. Ocular ultrasound. *Clin Rad* 1996; **51**: 533–544.

Kwong JS, Munk PL, Lin DTC, Vellet AD, Levin M, Buckley AR. Real-time sonography in ocular trauma. *AJR* 1992; **158**: 179–182.

McNicholas MMJ, Brophy DP, Power WJ, Griffin JF. Ocular sonography. *AJR* 1994; **163**: 921–926.

McNicholas MMJ, Power WJ, Griffin JF. Sonography in optic disk Drusen: Imaging findings and role in diagnosis when funduscopic findings are normal. *AJR* 1994; **162**: 161–163.

Munk PL, Vellet AD, Levin M, Lin DTC, Collyer RT. Sonography of the eye. *AJR* 1991; **157**: 1079–1086.

Ramji FG, Slovis TL, Baker JD. Orbital sonography in children. *Pediatr Radiol* 1996; **26**: 245–258.

Wong AD, Cooperberg PL, Ross WH, Araki DN Differentiation of detached retina and vitreous membrane with color flow Doppler. Radiology 1991; **178**: 429–431.

5

THE CHEST

Primary imaging of the chest is performed by chest X-ray. Ultrasound is a secondary imaging technique, used to supplement chest X-rays. Ultrasonic evaluation of the chest is impeded by the surrounding rib cage and air-filled lungs. It is usually performed in conjunction with other imaging techniques, e.g. chest X-ray, MRI or CT.

Ultrasound Technique

PREPARATION
None required.

TRANSDUCER
Type and frequency depends on the particular area of interest and patient build.

TECHNIQUE
This depends on the specific area of interest or pathology involved. For example, pleural effusions are best imaged subcostally or intercostally with the patient erect or in a decubitus position as fluid will collect in the dependent position. The ideal position of patient and choice of transducer will be given for each of the areas of interest covered in this chapter.

PLEURAL COLLECTIONS

Ultrasound can help to:

Determine the nature of a collection.

Distinguish between a mass-consolidation or an effusion.

Guide aspiration.

Determine whether simple tube or operative drainage of a collection is appropriate.

Types of fluid collection seen in childhood include:

Serous fluid: simple effusion

Pus. empyema

Blood: haemothorax

Chyle: chylothorax.

TECHNIQUE
Patient erect or lateral decubitus ideally, but prone or supine if the former is not possible. Suspended or quiet respiration.

Curvilinear transducer 5–7.5 MHz in infants and young children; 3.5 MHz in adolescents. The area of interest should be imaged in sequential longitudinal and transverse sections using both intercostal and subcostal approaches.

Simple pleural collections

CLINICAL PRESENTATION
Pneumonia.

Congestive heart failure.

Kidney disease e.g. glomerulonephritis, nephrotic syndrome.

Tumours.

Primary TB infections.

Pancreatitis.

The cause of an effusion in most children is infection.

ULTRASOUND APPEARANCES (Fig. 5.1)
- Hypo/anechoic fluid collection seen above the diaphragm.
- Examined erect, fluid tends to collect in the inferior pleural space.
- Large effusions may cause displacement of mediastinum and/or diaphragm.

NB. Tube aspiration is satisfactory for non-complicated effusions.

Empyema

CLINICAL PRESENTATION
Complication of pneumonia.

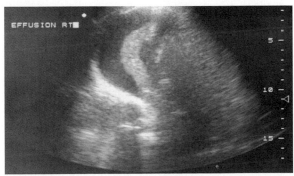

Figure 5.1 — An anechoic fluid collection above the right hemidiaphragm. The echogenic area within it is collapsed lung.

ULTRASOUND APPEARANCES (Fig. 5.2a and b)

● Anechoic/hypoechoic fluid collection.

● Numerous septae/strands.

● Echogenic debris.

● Appear more echoic as resolution occurs.

NB. More complex collections often require surgical drainage.

Haemothorax (Fig. 5.3)

CLINICAL PRESENTATION

Blunt abdominal/chest trauma.

Penetrating chest injury.

ULTRASOUND APPEARANCES

● Similar to empyema.

Chylothorax

CLINICAL PRESENTATION

Sometimes seen in the newborn.

Post-thoracotomy.

Following chest trauma.

ULTRASOUND APPEARANCES

● Similar to a simple effusion; the two cannot be distinguished ultrasonically.

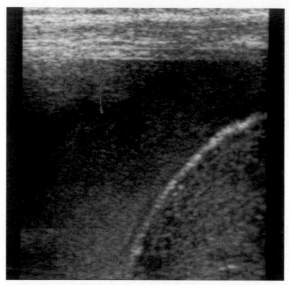

Figure 5.3 — Haemothorax a hypoechoic fluid collection, superior to the diaphragm, with echogenic debris suggesting a degree of organisation.

THE MEDIASTINUM

The space between the lungs and pleura which contains the heart and origins of the great vessels, part of the oesophagus, trachea, the vagus, phrenic and laryngeal nerves, lymph glands and vessels and thymus. In adults, the lungs may intervene between the mediastinum and chest wall preventing ultrasound access. In children, this is not usually a problem.

TECHNIQUE

Patient supine.

5–7.5 MHz curvilinear transducer for young children and infants.

3.5 MHz curvilinear transducer for adolescents.

Best imaged from suprasternal, intercostal and subxiphisternal approaches.

Thymus

Situated in the anterior mediastinum. Usually extends from the left brachiocephalic vein to the base of the aorta and superior vena cava (SVC).

The size varies, being large under 4 years of age and then gradually diminishing in size until it atrophies after puberty.

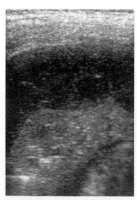

Figure 5.2 (a) — A mainly hypoechoic fluid collection with echogenic debris is seen displacing the atelectatic lung.

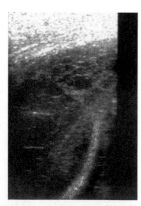

Figure 5.2 (b) — A complex multiloculated collection displaces the underlying lung.

Patients are usually referred for ultrasound following a chest X-ray with ? enlargd thymus. Ultrasound is used to distinguish between the normal thymus and a possible mediastinal mass.

CLINICAL PRESENTATION
Abnormal chest X-ray.

NORMAL ULTRASOUND APPEARANCES (Fig. 5.4)
- Variable shape
  - four sided structure < 5 years
  - more triangular > 5 years
  - rarely, extends into the neck.

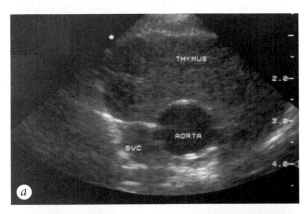

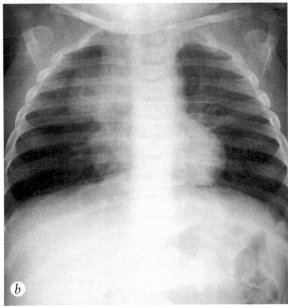

Figure 5.4 — (a) The normal thymus, homogeneous in echotexture, lying anterior to the aorta and superior vena cava. (b) Chest X-ray of same child.

- Homogeneous echotexture (similar to liver).
- Slightly less echogenic than liver/spleen.
- It lies in front of the great vessels.
- The normal thymus never compresses the great vessels.

PROBLEMS
The thymus becomes more difficult to image with increasing age due to its reduction in size and the air-filled lung in the anterior mediastinum.

Thymic abnormalities

Cysts

Rare.

ULTRASOUND APPEARANCES
- Anechoic well-defined lesions within the normal thymus which demonstrate posterior enhancement.
- +/- septations.

Tumours

Rare.

Lymphoma

Most common tumour involving the mediastinum.

CLINICAL PRESENTATION
Palpable nodal mass in the neck or supraclavicular region.

Breathlessness.

Symptoms of superior vena cava obstruction.

Widening of the anterior mediastinum on a chest X-ray.

ULTRASOUND APPEARANCES
- Solid well-defined mass.
- Homogeneous echotexture.
- Similar echogenicity to liver/spleen.
- May have an associated pleural effusion.

Teratoma

Usually a benign lesion.

CLINICAL PRESENTATION

Breathlessness.

Widening of the anterior mediastinum on a chest X-ray.

ULTRASOUND APPEARANCES (Fig. 5.5)
- Variable, may contain fat and calcification.
- Well-defined lesion.
- Multicystic/cystic lesion.
- Can be mainly solid.
- Often compresses the major vessels.

Pericardial effusion

Accumulation of fluid around the heart within the pericardial sac.

CLINICAL PRESENTATION

Symptoms of cardiac failure.

Shortness of breath.

Chest pain.

Enlarged heart on chest X-ray.

ULTRASOUND APPEARANCES (Fig. 5.6)
- Anechoic/hypoechoic fluid collection surrounding the heart.

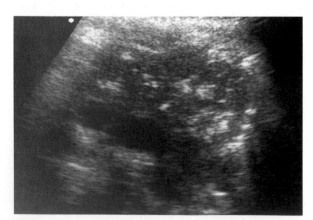

Figure 5.5 — An irregular-shaped mass, involving the thymus, containing echogenic foci representing areas of calcification.

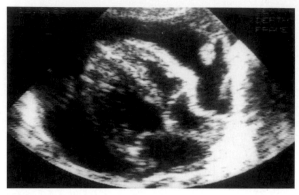

Figure 5.6 — Pericardial effusion, an anechoic fluid collection surrounding the heart.

- Mixed echogenicity with septae is seen when purulent.

Lymphadenopathy

Ultrasound can be used to detect lymphadenopathy in the mediastinal region.

Lymph nodes appear as well-defined masses, homogeneous in echotexture.

Mediastinal lymphangioma

Fluid-filled collection in the anterior chest.

May extend into the neck.

CLINICAL PRESENTATION

Neck or supraclavicular mass.

Increase in size usually indicates intralesional bleeding.

May compress vessels or trachea.

ULTRASOUND APPEARANCES
- Cystic collection often with septae.
- If complicated by bleeding, the fluid becomes echogenic.

TREATMENT

Aspiration of the fluid under ultrasound control with sclerotherapy is often undertaken.

THE DIAPHRAGM

The muscle which divides the chest and abdomen, responsible for breathing.

The purpose of ultrasound is:

To assess movement.

To detect disruption, e.g. diaphragmatic hernias or congenital weakness/thinness (eventration).

To detect subphrenic collections.

TECHNIQUE

Patient supine or in right and left lateral decubitus positions.

A curvilinear transducer, the frequency dependent on patient build.

The liver can be used as an acoustic window on the right and the spleen on the left, although the left is sometimes more difficult to image due to the stomach.

NORMAL ULTRASOUND APPERANCES (Figs. 5.7, 5.8)
Curved echogenic band between liver and diaphragm on the right and spleen and diaphragm on the left.

Assessment of movement

Movement of each hemidiaphragm is best assessed in a longitudinal section.

Paradoxical movement is best assessed by fluoroscopy. To assess using ultrasound, place the transducer in the midline and angle cranially. Both hemidiaphragms can be visualised on one image for comparison.

Causes of impairment of diaphragmatic movement include:

Large pleural effusions.

Subphrenic abscess.

Diaphragmatic hernia/eventration.

Inflammation.

Damage to the phrenic nerve after thoracic surgery.

Diaphragmatic hernia

Herniation of abdominal contents into the chest cavity through a defect in the diaphragm.

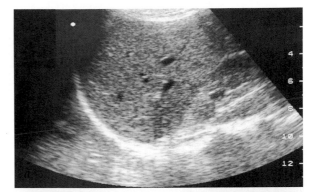

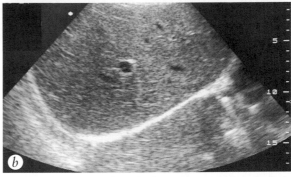

Figure 5.7 — The right hemidiaphragm is seen as an echogenic band superior to the liver in longitudinal section (a) and behind the liver in transverse section (b).

Most common type occurs on the left side posteriorly – Bochdalek; stomach, spleen, left kidney and bowel may all herniate through the defect.

May also occur on the right, usually anteriorly – Morgagni. Bowel with or without the liver herniates.

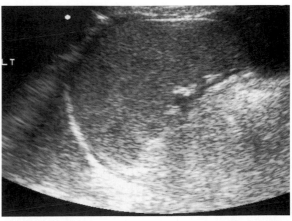

Figure 5.8 — The left hemidiaphragm, an echogenic band superior to the spleen; the air-filled lung obscures the diaphragm laterally.

Occlusion of the hepatic veins may result in Budd-Chiari malformation.

Hernias are usually isolated anomalies.

ASSOCIATED ANOMALIES:

Malrotation

Heart anomalies

Trisomy 18 + 21.

CLINICAL PRESENTATION

At birth

- tachypnoea

- dyspnoea

- cyanosis.

In older children

- may be asymptomatic, an incidental finding on chest X-ray

- vomiting

- dyspnoea

- mild epigastric pain.

ULTRASOUND APPEARANCES

- Disruption of the diaphragm, i.e. a loss or break in the normal echogenic line.

- Abdominal contents seen through the defect and within the chest, e.g. liver on right; spleen, left kidney, bowel on the left.

Eventration

Congenital weakness or thinness of the diaphragm which may be partial and affect only a portion.

Usually an isolated anomaly.

ASSOCIATED ANOMALIES:

Trisomy 13 + 18.

Pulmonary hyperplasia.

CLINICAL PRESENTATION

Usually of no clinical significance.

A large lesion may cause respiratory distress.

ULTRASOUND APPEARANCES (Fig. 5.9)

- Localised bulge in the diaphragm.

- Herniation of the liver/spleen into the chest cavity. May be difficult on ultrasound to differentiate from a hernia; continuity of the diaphragm, if demonstrated, distinguishes the two.

- Paradoxical movement of the weak diaphragmatic segment.

THE LUNGS

Normal aerated lung strongly reflects the ultrasound beam. Therefore abnormalities of the lungs can only be demonstrated if they are close to the chest wall, mediastinum or diaphragm.

Consolidation

A region of the lung acquires a semi-solid/solid consistency. (Air in the alveoli is replaced by inflammatory exudate.)

CLINICAL PRESENTATION

Pneumonia.

ULTRASOUND APPEARANCES (Fig. 5.10)

- Rarely defined.

- Hypoechoic in comparison to normal lung.

- May contain echogenic flecks caused by trapped air in the alveoli of the consolidated lung.

- Moves with respiration.

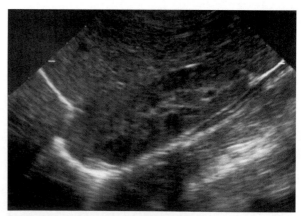

Figure 5.9 — Eventration: A longitudinal section of the right hemidiaphragm. The right kidney is shown herniating into the chest but the diaphragm remains intact.

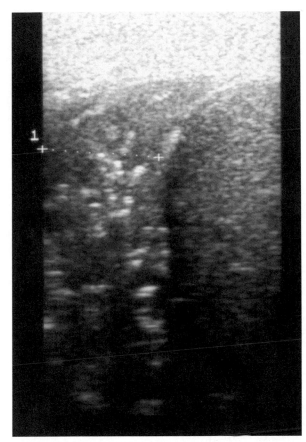

Figure 5.10 — The lung appears hypoechoic and contains echogenic foci, representing trapped air in the alveoli.

Lung abscess

A localised collection of pus in the lung tissues usually caused by infection with pyogenic material.

CAUSES

Pneumonia.

Pulmonary TB.

Obstruction of the bronchial tree (e.g. tumour, foreign body).

Inhalation of infected material (e.g. vomit or from a dental, nose or throat operation).

CLINICAL PRESENTATION

Rapid respiratory rate.

Fever.

ULTRASOUND APPEARANCES (Fig 5.11)

- Spherical/oval hypoechoic mass.
- Ill-defined, usually with a thick irregular wall.
- May demonstrate air–fluid level with the patient erect.
- May be single or multiple.
- Moves with respiration as it is intrapulmonary.

Lung cysts

Uncommon.

Acquired cysts can sometimes result from complications of pneumonia.

Congenital include:

Cystic adenomatoid malformation

Part of the normal lung parenchyma is replaced by cysts.

Three types:

Type I – one or more cysts > 2cm.

Type II – multiple smaller cysts.

Type III – tiny cysts resulting in a solid mass of tissue.

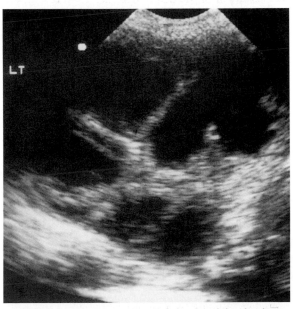

Figure 5.11 — Lung abscess. An ill-defined multiloculated mass consistent with an abscess.

CLINICAL PRESENTATION

Usually the diagnosis is made antenatally with post-natal follow-up.

May present at birth with respiratory distress.

ULTRASOUND APPEARANCES (Fig. 5.12)

Types I and II

- Complex mass of anechoic/hypoechoic lesions.
- Multiple septations.
- Echogenic foci which cast acoustic shadows if the cysts contain air.

Type III

- A solid echogenic mass.

NB. Colour flow imaging should be performed to differentiate the lesion from an arteriovenous malformation (Types I and II) or pulmonary sequestration (Type III) and ensure no vascular supply.

Bronchogenic cyst

Rare developmental abnormality.

Ultrasound is useful only if the cyst is located close to the chest wall.

CLINICAL PRESENTATION

Respiratory distress.

Signs of infection.

Often incidental finding on chest X-ray.

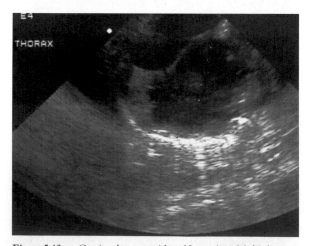

Figure 5.12 — Cystic adenomatoid malformation. Multiple cysts of < 2cm, consistent with cystic adenomatoid malformation Type II.

ULTRASOUND APPEARANCES (Fig. 5.13)

- Hypoechoic.
- Usually thin walled; however, sometimes thick walled especially if infected.
- Complex cysts contain fluid and air, appear hypoechoic with echogenic contents.

NB. If thick walled, must be investigated to differentiate from pulmonary cystic mesenchymal hamartoma which has a malignant tendency.

Pulmonary sequestration

A mass of non-functioning lung tissue which has abnormal communication with the bronchial tree or pulmonary vessels and is supplied by an anomalous vessel usually arising from the aorta. The diagnosis is often made on antenatal scans, the child being asymptomatic at birth.

Intralobar

Occurs within the visceral pleura of an otherwise normal lung.

Most common type.

Diagnosed usually < 20 years.

CLINICAL PRESENTATION

Recurrent pneumonia, usually lower lobe.

Extralobar

The sequestrated lung has a separate pleural lining.

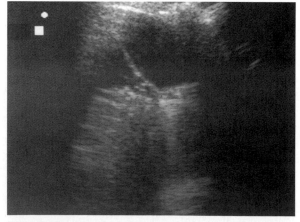

Figure 5.13 — Bronchogenic cyst. A thin-walled anechoic lesion is demonstrated close to the chest wall within the left lung.

Diagnosed usually in infancy (< 6 months).

More common in males and on the left side.

Associated with pleural effusions.

ASSOCIATED ANOMALIES
Cystic adenomatoid malformation

Bochdalek hernia.

CLINICAL PRESENTATION
Dyspnoea.

Cyanosis.

ULTRASOUND APPEARANCES (Fig. 5.14)
- Variable, depends on aeration of the sequestered lung.
- A sequestration that communicates with the bronchial tree appears echogenic and, as it contains air, reverberation artefact is seen.
- A sequestration that does not communicate with the bronchial tree appears as a solid, homogeneous, echogenic mass, usually posteriorly within the lower lobe.
- Colour flow imaging may help to determine anomalous feeding vessels (the presence of which allows it to be distinguished from cystic adenomatoid malformation).

NB. MRI is usually performed to confirm ultrasonic diagnosis.

Lung tumours

Primary lung tumours are rare. Types include leiomyosarcoma, rhabdomyosarcoma and bronchogenic carcinoma.

Pulmonary metastases are the commonest cause of lung malignancy in children.

CLINICAL PRESENTATION
Fever.

Cough.

Worsening dyspnoea.

Mass on chest X-ray.

ULTRASOUND APPEARANCES (Fig. 5.15)
- The position of the mass will influence whether it is accessible to imaging with ultrasound. A peripherally placed mass can easily be imaged.
- Mass of variable size.
- Solid/Cystic.
- Usually well-defined.
- May exert a mass effect on adjacent structures.

THE CHEST WALL

Formed of the rib cage, intercostal muscles and the chest wall muscles.

Easily accessible to ultrasound assessment.

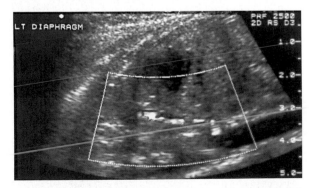

Figure 5.14 — An echogenic mass is demonstrated close to the left hemidiaphragm which contains cystic lesions. The anomalous feeding vessel seen arising from the aorta distinguishes it from cystic adenomatoid malformation.

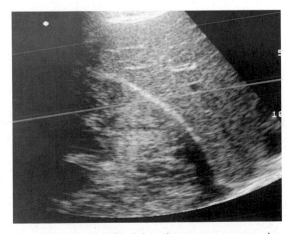

Figure 5.15 — A well-defined, large heterogeneous mass, above the diaphragm, displacing the liver inferiorly.

TRANSDUCER

High frequency linear array.

TECHNIQUE

Supine. Patient comfortable.

Always examine normal contralateral side.

CLINICAL INDICATIONS

Lumps.

Asymmetry.

Rib cage

Swellings at the costochondral junctions causing either a local lump or asymmetry are a common cause for concern. They are usually painless.

CAUSE

Usually unknown.

Post-traumatic.

Post inflammatory.

Infection – very rare.

ULTRASOUND APPEARANCES

- Normal ribs: anterior surface of the rib appears echogenic with posterior acoustic shadowing.

- Normal costochondral junctions: more superficial than the rib and hypoechoic.

- Costochondral lesions: also hypoechoic but have increased thickness compared with normal side.

Rib tumours

Include:

Ewing's sarcoma.

Primitive neuroectodermal tumour.

Both at presentation usually have a large soft tissue mass extending extrapleurally with an associated large pleural effusion.

ULTRASOUND APPEARANCES

- Large solid hypoechoic mass.

- If necrotic, may be mixed solid or cystic.

- May contain calcification.

- Rib destruction may be visible.

- Periosteal reaction on rib may be visible.

- Underlying effusion is often haemorrhagic.

PITFALL

Necrotic tumour may appear solid. Cannot be distinguished from viable tumour tissue.

If ultrasound-guided biopsy using extrapleural approach is employed prior imaging with CT should be done to identify areas of non-necrotic tumour.

Rib cage infection

Rare.

Usual presentation chest wall mass or abscess.

ULTRASOUND APPEARANCES

- Abscess mass – hypoechoic.

- May contain central necrosis.

- Periosteal reaction on rib may be visible.

BREAST ULTRASOUND

Mammography is not performed in young girls and ultrasound is more valuable in examining young dense glandular breasts.

PREPARATION

None required.

TRANSDUCER

High frequency linear transducer, e.g. 10 MHz.

TECHNIQUE

Supine, or rotated slightly onto the unaffected side with the arm of affected side raised above the head. The breast is scanned in a clockwise fashion using the nipple as a reference point. Both breasts are scanned for comparison.

If there is a palpable lump it may be necessary to hold it in a fixed position to enable adequate assessment.

Normal appearances of breast

The breast appears hyperechoic and heterogeneous in echotexture (Fig. 5.16).

Post puberty: normal ductular tissue as for adults.

INDICATIONS FOR BREAST ULTRASOUND IN CHILDREN

A palpable mass – to determine the nature, i.e. cystic/solid.

Guided aspiration.

Breast asymmetry.

Painful breast – exclusion of a mass.

Cysts

CLINICAL PRESENTATION

Palpable mass.

Pain.

ULTRASOUND APPEARANCES (Fig. 5.17)
- Well defined, with smooth walls.

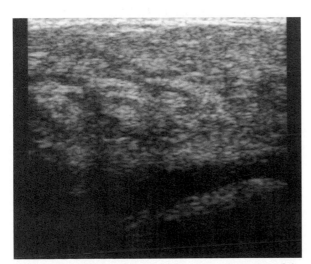

Figure 5.16 — Hyperechoic, heterogeneous echotexture of the glandular tissue of the normal breast.

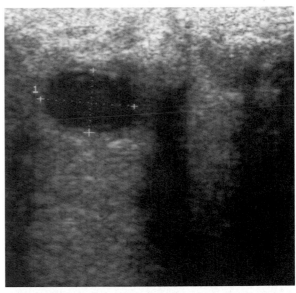

Figure 5.17 — A thin-walled, well-defined anechoic lesion which demonstrates post-cystic enhancement within the normal glandular tissue of the breast.

- Anechoic.
- Demonstrate post cystic enhancement.
- Usually solitary.
- May contain septae.

Abscess

CLINICAL PRESENTATION

Palpable mass.

Pain.

Tender to touch.

Skin red and hot over the mass.

ULTRASOUND APPEARANCES (Fig. 5.18)
- Hypoechoic – contain echogenic debris.
- Thickened and irregular walls.
- May demonstrate fluid/debris level.
- Septae.
- More commonly occur in the periareolar area.
- Cystic enhancement.

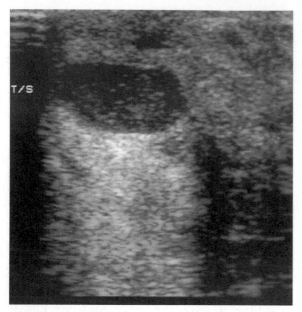

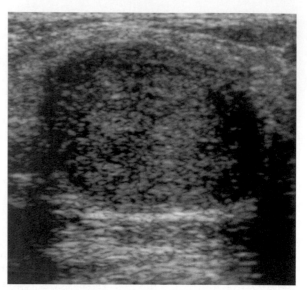

Figure 5.18 — A thick-walled lesion which is mainly hypoechoic, although some echoes are demonstrated within it. Note the cystic enhancement posteriorly to the lesion.

Figure 5.19 — A well-defined hypoechoic lesion, homogeneous in echotexture. NB. No cystic enhancement.

Fibroadenoma

The most common breast mass found in children.

CLINICAL PRESENTATION
Palpable mass.

Pain.

ULTRASOUND APPEARANCES (Fig. 5.19)
- Well defined.
- Oval in shape.
- Hypoechoic.
- Homogeneous echotexture.
- Demonstrate no enhancement.
- Variable in size.
- May be multiple.

NB. Malignant lesions in children are very rare but lymphoma and rhabdomyosarcoma occur and cannot be distinguished from fibroadenoma by ultrasound.

Breast asymmetry

Ultrasound is performed to confirm the presence of normal breast tissue and rule out the possibility of a mass.

CLINICAL PRESENTATION (Fig. 5.20)
A visible/palpable difference in the size of the breasts.

ULTRASOUND APPEARANCES
- Normal breast tissue is identified.
- Difference in size.

Breast tumours

Rare.

Most common lesion, cystosarcoma phalloides, a benign tumour which occurs in adolescents (16–19 years) and is difficult to distinguish on ultrasound from fibroadenoma.

Breast carcinoma is very rare under 20 years of age.

Most common malignancy is due to metastases, from a primary malignancy such as lymphoma, leukaemia, rhabdomyosarcoma or neuroblastoma.

Lymphoma and rhabdomyosarcoma may present primarily in the breast.

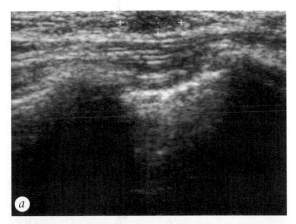

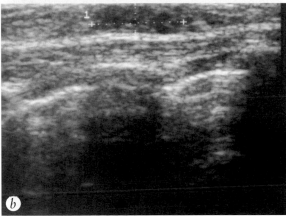

Figure 5.20 a, b — Normal prepubertal breast tissue is demonstrated in a 3-year-old girl. Note the difference in size between the breast buds in longitudinal section.

CLINICAL PRESENTATION

Breast asymmetry.

A palpable mass in the breast.

Palpable axillary nodes.

Pain is infrequent.

ULTRASOUND APPEARANCES

● A solid well defined lesion.

● Infiltration appears as irregularity of texture in comparison to the contralateral side (Fig. 5.21).

Further reading

Adam EJ, Ignotus PI. Sonography of the thymus in healthy children: frequency of visualization, size, and appearance. *AJR* 1993; **161**: 153–155.

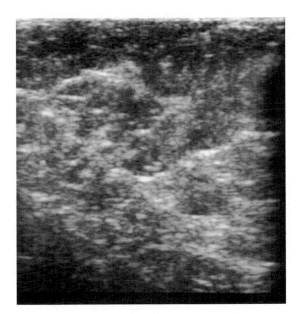

Figure 5.21 — Irregularity in the echotexture of the left breast consistent with lymphoma infiltration.

Amodio J, Abramson S, Berdon W, Stolar C, Markowitz R, Kasznica J. Iatrogenic causes of large pleural effusions in the premature infant: ultrasonic and radiographic findings. *Pediatr Radiol* 1987; **17**: 104–108.

Boothroyd A, Carty H. Breast masses in childhood and adolescence; a presentation of 17 cases and a review of the literature. *Pediatr Radiol* 1994; **24**: 81–84.

Carty H. Ultrasound of the normal thymus in the infant: a simple method of resolving a clinical dilemma. *BJR* 1990; **63**: 737–738.

Erasmie U, Lundell B. Pulmonary lesions mimicking pericardial effusion on ultrasonography. *Pediatr Radiol* 1987; **17**: 447–450.

Felker RE, Tonkin ILD. Imaging of pulmonary sequestration. *AJR* 1990; **154**: 241–249.

Goldstein DP, Miller V. Breast masses in adolescent females. *Clin Pediatr* 1982; **21**: 17–19.

Haller JO, Schneider M, Kassner EG, Friedman AP, Waldroup LD. Sonographic evaluation of the chest in infants and children. *AJR* 1980; **134**: 1019–1027.

Han BK, Babcock DS, Oestreich AE. The normal thymus in infancy: sonographic characteristics. *Radiology* 1989; **170**: 471–474.

Hartenberg MA, Brewer WH. Cystic adenomatoid malformation of the lung: identification by sonography. *AJR* 1983; **140**: 693–694.

Hernanz–Schulman M, Stein SM, Neblett WW, et al. Pulmonary sequestration: diagnosis with colour Doppler sonography and a new theory of associated hydrothorax. *Radiology* 1991; **180**: 817–821.

Kaude JV, Laurin S. Ultrasonographic demonstration of systemic artery feeding extrapulmonary sequestration. *Pediatr Radiol* 1984; **14**: 226–227.

King RM, Telander RL, Smithson WA, Banks PM, Han MT. Primary mediastinal tumours in children. *J Pediatr Surg* 1982; **17**: 512–520.

Laing IA, Teel RL, Stark AR. Diaphragmatic movement in new–born infants. *J Pediatr* 1988; **112**: 638–643.

McLoud TC, Flower CDR. Imaging the pleural: sonography CT and MR imaging. *AJR* 1991; **156**: 1145–1153.

Moccia WA, Kaude JV, Felman AH. Congenital eventration of the diaphragm. Diagnosis by ultrasound. *Pediatr Radiol* 1981; **10**: 197–200.

O'Laughlin MP, Huhta JC, Murphy DJ. Ultrasound examination of extracardiac chest masses in children. *J Ultrasound Med* 1987; **6**: 151–157.

Rogers DA, Lobe TE, Rao BN, Fleming ID, Schropp KP, Pratt CB, Pappa AS. Breast malignancy in children. *J Pediatr Surg* 1994; **29**: 52–55.

Rosado-de-Christenson ML, Stocker JT. Congenital cystic adenomatoid malformation. *Radiographics* 1991; **11**: 865–886.

Rudick MG, Wood BP. The use of ultrasound in the diagnosis of a large thymic cyst. *Pediatr Radiol* 1980; **10**: 113–115.

Targhetta R, Chavagneux R, Bourgeois JM, Dauzat M, Balmes P, Pourcelot L. Sonographic approach to diagnosing pulmonary consolidation. *J Ultrasound Med* 1992; **11**: 667–672.

Wernecke K, Vassallo P, Pötter R, Lückener HG, Peters PE. Mediastinal tumours: sensitivity of detection with sonography compared with CT and radiography. *Radiology* 1990; **175**: 137–143.

West MS, Donaldson JS, Shkolnik A. Pulmonary sequestration: diagnosis by ultrasound. *J Ultrasound Med* 1989; **8**: 125–129.

Worthen NJ, Worthen WF. Disruption of the diaphragmatic echoes: a sonographic sign of diaphragmatic disease. *J Clin Ultrasound* 1982; **10**: 43–45.

Yang PC, Luh KT, Chang DB, Wu HD, Yu CJ, Kuo SH. Value of sonography in determining the nature of pleural effusion: analysis of 320 cases. *AJR* 1992; **159**: 29–33.

Yang PC, Luh KT, Lee YC, Chang DB, Yu CC, Wu HD, Lee LN. Lung abscesses: US examination and US-guided transthoracic aspiration. *Radiology* 1991; **180**: 171–175.

Yeh HC, Halton KP, Gray CE. Anatomic variations and abnormalities in the diaphragm seen with US. *Radiographics* 1990; **10**: 1019–1030.

Zangwill BC, Stocker JT. Congenital cystic adenomatoid malformation within an extralobar pulmonary sequestration. *Pediatr Pathol* 1993; **13**: 309–315.

6

THE GASTROINTESTINAL TRACT

Pyloric stenosis

There is abnormal thickening of the circular muscle of the pylorus, which elongates and constricts the pyloric canal.

Cause: unknown.

Age range: 2–8 weeks.

Peak incidence: 5–6 weeks.

More common in boys.

Incidence: 3 in 1000.

Familial pattern.

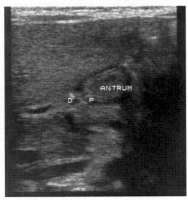

Figure 6.1 — Normal calibre pylorus opening into the first part of the duodenum.

CLINICAL PRESENTATION

Projectile, non-bilious vomiting (positive test feed).

Palpable olive-shaped epigastric mass. Can be felt in approximately 80% of affected children.

Failure to thrive.

Exaggerated gastric peristalsis visible through the abdominal wall.

CHOICE OF TRANSDUCER

10 MHz linear transducer.

PATIENT PREPARATION

None.

TECHNIQUE

The pylorus is usually identified by locating the gallbladder and moving the transducer medially towards the patient's midline or by finding the stomach and following it to the antrum and therefore the pylorus (Fig. 6.1). If the patient has this condition then the thickened muscle will usually be imaged immediately. If difficulty is experienced with the patient supine, the right side down decubitus position should be used: fluid fills the antrum allowing visualisation of the pyloric canal. If there is insufficient fluid in the stomach, fluid can be given orally.

NB. The antrum of the stomach should be watched in real-time for opening and for motility. If the stomach contents are seen to pass through the canal from the stomach then this is unlikely to represent pyloric stenosis.

ULTRASOUND APPEARANCES

- Thickened outer hypoechoic muscle with an inner echogenic layer representing mucosa and submucosa, and a central anechoic canal. (Fig. 6.2a,b).

- Measurements of the hypertrophied pyloric muscle are most reliably obtained on a longitudinal section ('hamburger' sign).

- A canal length of ≥ 16 mm and a single muscle thickness of > 3 mm is diagnostic of pyloric stenosis. (Fig. 6.3).

- Failure of the pyloric canal to open with a peristaltic wave.

PITFALLS

The size of the pyloric muscle is related to the patient's age and weight. Criteria appropriate for term infants may not be appropriate for premature infants.

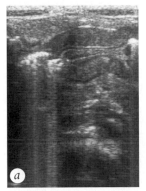 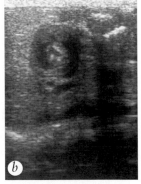

Figures 6.2 — Longitudinal (a) and transverse (b) sections illustrating pyloric stenosis. The outer hypoechoic muscle is thickened.

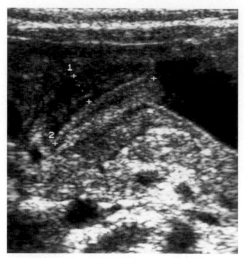

Figure 6.3 — Pyloric stenosis; hypoechoic muscle wall thickness of 4.6 mm (1), and a canal length of 19 mm (2).

If the pylorus appears thickened but does not fit the measurement criteria, then repeat scan in 24 hours, as the condition can develop over a few days.

Imaging the pylorus tangentially will give erroneous measurements.

Measurements of the pylorus should only include muscle thickness and not mucosa and/or pyloric canal.

ASSOCIATED ANOMALIES

Occasionally renal anomalies, e.g. duplex, obstruction, horseshoe kidney.

TREATMENT

Pyloromyotomy which involves splitting of the muscle.

Intussusception

Occurs in young children usually under two.

Cause uncertain but is thought to be related to viral illness in which there is enlargement of the Peyer's patches within the bowel.

May be caused by Meckel's diverticulum or polyp acting as a lead point.

A segment of bowel telescopes into another.

Four varieties are described: the commonest is ileo-colic intussusception. Other varieties are colo-colic, ileo-ileo-colic and ileo-ileal intussusception.

The disease is equally common in boys and girls.

Known complication of cystic fibrosis.

CLINICAL PRESENTATION

Colicky abdominal pain.

The child draws their legs up and goes white during the attack.

In 30% of patients there may be a 'redcurrant jelly' stool.

Many children simply present with colicky abdominal pain, without any stool abnormality.

A typical length of history is between twelve and twenty-four hours.

Palpable abdominal mass in about 50% of patients.

CHOICE OF TRANSDUCER

10 MHz linear transducer supplemented by a curvilinear to examine the pelvis.

PATIENT PREPARATION

None as the patient presents as an emergency case.

ULTRASOUND APPEARANCES

• The intussuscipiens is usually located in the right upper quadrant (RUQ).

• May also be seen in the transverse colon, or splenic flexure.

• A typical appearance in transverse section is described as a target or doughnut sign.

• The different layers of bowel are seen with the bowel wall being hypoechoic and bowel mucosa and serosa appearing echogenic (Fig. 6.4).

• In longitudinal section, the intussusception has a reniform appearance.

• Small amounts of free fluid between the bowel loops is a common finding.

• A large amount of free intraperitoneal fluid implies extensive bowel oedema and potentially impending infarction and is a contraindication to hydrostatic reduction.

• Colour flow imaging can be used to confirm blood flow in viable bowel (Fig. 6.5) with absence of blood flow suggesting infarcted, gangrenous bowel.

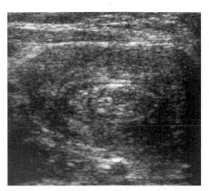

Figure 6.4 — Target lesion in transverse section diagnostic of intussusception. Hypoechoic bowel wall and echogenic bowel mucosa and serosa.

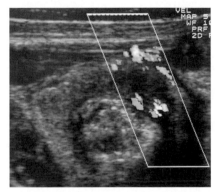

Figure 6.5 — Colour flow imaging confirming blood flow within viable bowel. Note small amount of free fluid around bowel loops.

PITFALLS

If the child's abdomen is very gassy, due to bowel obstruction, direct scanning through the central abdominal wall may prove impossible.

Scanning laterally, with the probe angled under the bowel gas, may render a lesion visible, not detectable with direct scanning.

DIFFERENTIAL DIAGNOSIS

If no intussusception is demonstrated on ultrasound, a likely alternative diagnosis is mesenteric adenitis. A search of the mesentery for enlarged lymph nodes may help to make a positive diagnosis of this condition and will prevent unnecessary surgery.

TREATMENT

Hydrostatic or pneumatic reduction can be successful; otherwise surgical reduction and resection.

Malrotation and volvulus

Malrotation is a congenital abnormality with failure during embryonic development of normal rotation of all or part of the bowel. The mesenteric pedicle is narrowed and the duodenojejunal junction is abnormally positioned. Instead of lying to the left of the spine posteriorly, it is found to the right of the spine anteriorly.

There is a predisposition for twisting of bowel to occur (volvulus) due to the narrowed mesenteric pedicle. The SMA and SMV, which are contained within the pedicle, can occlude, causing ischaemia and infarction of bowel.

CLINICAL PRESENTATION

Bilious vomiting.

Abdominal pain.

Abdominal distension if the bowel is compromised.

ULTRASOUND APPEARANCES

Malrotation

- Fluid-filled 1st and 2nd parts of the duodenum to the right of the spine.

- Demonstration of reversal of the normal relationship between the SMA and SMV. (Fig. 6.6a,b)

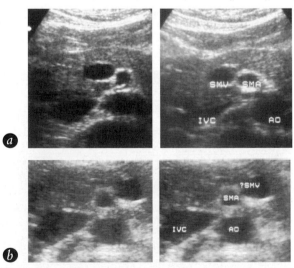

Figure 6.6 — Transverse sections demonstrating (a) normal relationship of the SMA and SMV and (b) reversal of the normal relationship of the SMA and SMV; the SMV lying to the left of the SMA.

- If the vein lies anterior or to the left of the artery this may suggest malrotation. However, vessel inversion can occur in patients with normal midgut rotation and conversely can be absent in patients with malrotation.

Volvulus

- A mass of twisted bowel loops with thickened echogenic bowel wall (haemorrhage and oedema) (Fig. 6.7).

- Whirlpool sign may be seen on colour flow due to the spiralling of the SMA.

- Free fluid in the peritoneum.

- Pulsating SMA.

ASSOCIATED ANOMALIES

Omphalocele.

Gastroschisis.

Diaphragmatic hernia.

Duodenal atresia.

Duodenal web.

NB. Malrotation is a life threatening condition. Not all children with malrotation have abnormal position of the SMA/SMV. Any child suspected of malrotation should have urgent upper GI contrast studies.

Obstruction and ileus

Small bowel obstruction

Can be as a result of atresia of the duodenum, ileum or jejunum, malrotation, meconium ileus or intussusception, or postoperative adhesions.

ULTRASOUND APPEARANCES

- Dilated fluid-filled loops of bowel with increased activity (Fig. 6.8). However, these findings are non-specific and can be seen with gastroenteritis.

- Some ascites may be present (anechoic serous fluid in the peritoneal cavity).

- Presence of unsuspected mass if this is the cause of obstruction.

Ileus

Mechanical, dynamic or adynamic obstruction of the bowel.

CLINICAL PRESENTATION

Pain.

Abdominal distension.

Vomiting.

Absence of passage of stool and bowel sound.

Fever, dehydration.

ULTRASOUND APPEARANCES

- Dilated fluid-filled loops of bowel with decreased activity.

- Bowel content can appear echogenic.

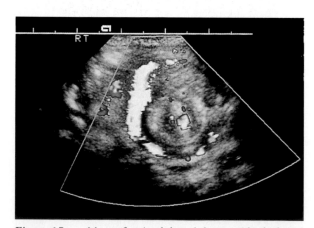

Figure 6.7 — Mass of twisted bowel loops with thickened echogenic bowel wall in a 3-week-old baby. Colour flow illustrates the spiral appearance of the superior mesenteric artery.

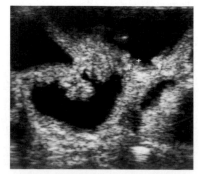

Figure 6.8 — Dilated fluid-filled loops of bowel in 11-month-old girl with small bowel obstruction. The bowel wall is normal: 24 mm.

Bowel wall thickening

Crohn's disease

Inflammatory bowel condition most commonly affecting the terminal ileum.

Cause unknown.

May affect any part of the bowel.

CLINICAL PRESENTATION

Abdominal pain.

Diarrhoea.

Anaemia.

Lethargy.

Growth failure.

Aphthous ulcers.

ULTRASOUND APPEARANCES

- Hypoechoic, thickened bowel wall surrounding an echogenic centre of compressed mucosa and/or intraluminal air (Fig. 6.9).
- Peristalsis is reduced.
- Abscess – hypoechoic or complex mass.
- Enlarged lymph nodes.
- Colour flow will demonstrate hypervascularity of the affected bowel.

OTHER INVESTIGATIONS

Endoscopy.

Contrast studies.

TREATMENT

Mainly conservative with medical and dietary management.

Surgery if obstruction develops.

Cystic fibrosis

A congenital metabolic disorder in which secretions of exocrine glands are abnormal. Excessive mucus causes obstruction of passageways including the intestines. There is malabsorption throughout the bowel.

ULTRASOUND APPEARANCES

- Thickened bowel wall, fluid-filled or echogenic mucosa (Fig. 6.10a,b).

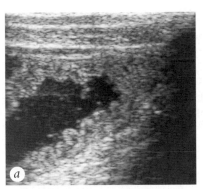
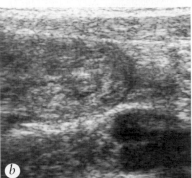

Figure 6.10 — Cystic fibrosis; longitudinal section showing thickened bowel wall with fluid-filled lumen (a) or echogenic mucosa (b).

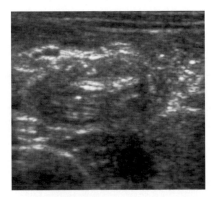

Figure 6.9 — Crohn's disease; transverse section showing hypoechoic, thickened bowel wall surrounding an echogenic centre of compressed mucosa.

- Intussusception.
- Transient intussusceptions may be seen.
- Gallstones.
- Hyperechoic pancreas.

Henoch-Schönlein purpura

An idiopathic systemic vasculitis.

CLINICAL PRESENTATION
Purpura, abdominal pain due to haemorrhage and / or oedema of the GIT.

ULTRASOUND APPEARANCES
- Hypoechoic bowel wall thickening (Fig. 6.11).
- Colour flow imaging may show hypervascularity in the mucosa and bowel wall.
- Intussusception can be an added complication.

Typhlitis

Inflammation of the caecum occurs in patients on chemotherapy most frequently with leukaemia. It affects the right colon.

ULTRASOUND APPEARANCES
- Thickened hypoechoic bowel wall, echogenic mucosa.
- Decreased or absent peristalsis.
- Colour flow imaging may demonstrate hypervascularity of both the mucosa and bowel wall.

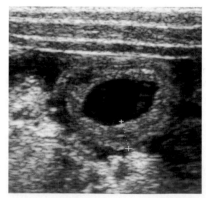

Figure 6.11 — Henoch-Schönlein purpura; transverse section showing oedematous thickened bowel wall due to haemorrhage.

Mesenteric adenitis

Inflammation of a mesenteric lymph node(s).

CLINICAL PRESENTATION
Acute abdominal pain.

ULTRASOUND APPEARANCES
- Multiple, enlarged, hypoechoic mesenteric lymph nodes (> 5 mm in diameter) (Fig. 6.12).
- May be bowel wall thickening (> 3 mm when bowel is distended).
- Nodes will not demonstrate blood flow on colour imaging.

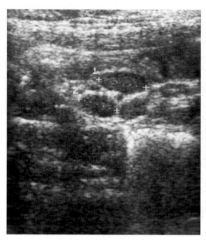

Figure 6.12 — Multiple enlarged hypoechoic mesenteric lymph nodes greater than 5 mm in diameter.

Duplication cyst

Congenital anomaly that contains intestinal mucosa and smooth muscle. It is located on the mesenteric border of the bowel.

Most are found in the distal ileum but other sites include the distal oesophagus, stomach and duodenum.

CLINICAL PRESENTATION
Vomiting (secondary to bowel obstruction).

Abdominal pain.

Asymptomatic abdominal mass.

ULTRASOUND APPEARANCES

- Well-defined, usually unilocular.

- An- or hypoechoic mass with posterior cystic enhancement.

- Can be echogenic with septa due to haemorrhage.

- Cyst has echogenic inner lining (mucosa) and a surrounding hypoechoic rim (muscle wall).

- The presence of these two layers (Fig. 6.13) helps to exclude other cystic masses such as mesenteric or omental cyst, choledochal cyst, ovarian cyst, pancreatic pseudocyst and abscess.

- Meckel's diverticulum can have a similar appearance to a duplication cyst.

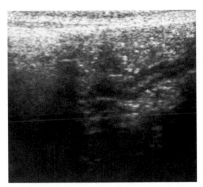

Figure 6.14 — Normal appendix demonstrating a thin echogenic lining with a hypoechoic wall, and a diameter of less than 6 mm.

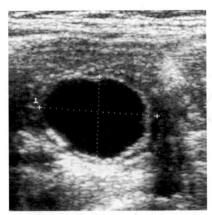

Figure 6.13 — Anechoic, well-defined cyst with posterior cystic enhancement. Note the presence of two layers: echogenic inner lining (mucosa) and hypoechoic rim (muscle wall).

Appendix

Normal appendix

ULTRASOUND APPEARANCES

- Seen infrequently using ultrasound but when visualised it appears as a blind-ended tubular structure on longitudinal sections.

- It has a thin, echogenic lining, hypoechoic wall and tapered end, and may be slightly compressible.

- Its maximum outer diameter should be less than 6 mm (Fig. 6.14). Length is irrelevant.

- No demonstrable blood flow on colour imaging.

Appendicitis

Appendicitis is due to obstruction of the appendix lumen by faeces or a faecolith. The vascular supply to the appendix is by end-arteries which, once thrombosed, will lead to gangrene followed by perforation.

The acute inflammation may resolve if the obstruction is relieved but a further attack is likely.

More often, the inflamed appendix undergoes gangrene and then perforates, either with a localised appendix abscess or general peritonitis. Rare complications are subphrenic abscess, portal vein thrombosis and liver abscess.

The most common cause of an acute surgical abdomen in childhood occurs between 6 and 12 years of age.

CLINICAL PRESENTATION

High temperature and increased pulse rate.

Localised pain, tenderness and rigidity on palpation in the RIF.

Pain commences as a central, peri-umbilical colic which moves to the RIF or more accurately to the site of the inflamed appendix. The pain is aggravated by movement and the patient prefers to lie still with knees flexed.

Nausea and vomiting.

Anorexia.

Constipation/diarrhoea – usually due to a pelvic abscess.

Tender and rigid abdomen with absent bowel sounds indicating peritonitis and ileus.

PATIENT PREPARATION

None as patient presents as an emergency examination.

TRANSDUCER

Linear 10 MHz to show the appendix, bowel movement and local RIF structures. The rest of the abdomen – especially pelvis and subphrenic spaces – may need a 3–5 MHz curved transducer examination.

PATIENT POSITION

Supine.

TECHNIQUE

Ask the patient to point to the site of pain with one finger. Scanning this area may result in rapid identification of the appendix, thereby shortening the examination time and decreasing associated patient discomfort. It is also helpful in identifying an aberrantly located appendix.

The transducer is placed in transverse section superior to the level of the umbilicus and continued caudally in the RIF. The colon with its hypoechoic muscle wall and inner echogenic mucosa, iliopsoas muscle and iliac vessels can be identified. The inflamed appendix usually is visualised at the base of the caecal tip. Gentle pressure should be applied to the abdomen by the transducer and the compressibility of the appendix noted. A normal appendix will be slightly compressible, an inflamed appendix will be non-compressible. The transducer is then rotated through 90 degrees and longitudinal sections are obtained. Again, compression should be applied and the compressibility noted.

In addition to scanning anteriorly over the right lower quadrant, if very gassy it may be useful to scan laterally in the right flank as occasionally a retro-caecal appendix can only be visualised by doing this.

ULTRASOUND APPEARANCES

- The lumen of the inflamed appendix is usually fluid-filled and may have echogenic foci with distal acoustic shadowing which represents intraluminal gas or solid material such as faeces or appendicolith (Fig. 6.15).

- Its diameter measured from the outside wall to outside wall is greater than 6 mm.

- On transverse section, the appendix can appear as a target lesion (Fig. 6.16). The fluid-filled lumen is surrounded by echogenic mucosa and then the hypoechoic bowel wall (Fig. 6.17).

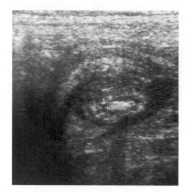

Figure 6.15 — Transverse section of an inflamed appendix demonstrating an appendicolith, displaying acoustic shadowing.

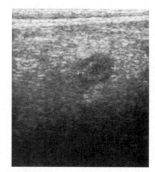

Figure 6.16 — Transverse section of an inflamed appendix appearing as a target lesion.

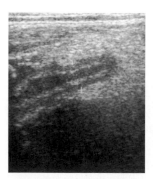
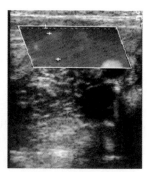

Figure 6.17 — Longitudinal section of an inflamed appendix illustrating a fluid-filled lumen, echogenic mucosa and hypoechoic bowel wall.

Figure 6.18 — Power Doppler of an inflamed appendix demonstrating hyperaemia of the bowel wall, and a fluid-filled lumen.

- Localised ileus with diminished or no bowel movement is frequent.

- A small amount of peri-appendiceal fluid may be seen. Lymphadenopathy is present in the adjacent mesentery in 30% of cases.

- On colour imaging, hyperperfusion of blood vessels at the periphery of the inflamed appendix can be demonstrated (Fig. 6.18).

Perforated appendix

ULTRASOUND APPEARANCES

- Dilated appendix with hypoechoic lumen and irregular walls.

- Peri-caecal fluid collection may be present.

- Non visualisation of the echogenic mucosa of the appendix.

The major complications of perforated appendix are abscess formation and peritonitis.

Abscess formation

Variable appearances; may be an-, hypo-, or hyperechoic or complex with both hypo- and hyperechoic areas, depending on the stage examined.

NB. A fluid collection does not always indicate perforation but may be a response to inflammation. In girls, it may be difficult to separate an appendiceal abscess from an ovarian process such as tubo-ovarian abscess (in appropriate age group).

Peritonitis

Dilated bowel loops with thick echogenic walls.

Ascites.

Mucocele of the appendix

Due to chronic obstruction with build up of luminal secretions.

History of recurrent RIF pain.

ULTRASOUND APPEARANCES

Fluid-filled structure in the RIF.

TREATMENT

Acute appendicitis: surgery.

Advanced peritonitis: surgery (i.e. abscess drainage +/- peritoneal lavage).

Antibiotics.

Recurrent attacks: elective surgery if the diagnosis is accurate.

Post appendicectomy

Infected fluid collections are commonly demonstrated early postoperatively and most will be located in the pelvis. Such fluid collections are treated with antibiotics and typically resolve in several weeks or months (Fig. 6.19).

ULTRASOUND APPEARANCES

- Variable appearances depending on its age.

- Can appear as solid mass early on but as liquefication occurs can be mixed echoes; cystic with echogenic areas representing infection (Fig. 6.20), fluid level, septations (Fig. 6.21).

- Variable in shape as conforms to intraperitoneal compartments.

- May also get wound abscess or seroma; both are seen as a variable echo collection under the wound.

MERITS

With experience, the accuracy is 93%.

LIMITATIONS

Difficult to perform if the patient is gassy or the appendix is retrocaecal.

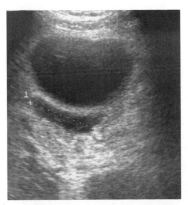

Figure 6.19 — Fluid collection behind the bladder representing a small pelvic collection three days post appendicectomy.

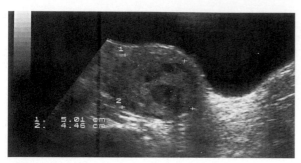

Figure 6.20 — Right adnexal mass of mixed echogenicity post appendicectomy. In this 11-year-old girl the right ovary was positively identified and was normal.

Difficult to perform if inexperienced.

Fairly time-consuming examination.

Non diagnostic if patient is obese.

Small percentage of patients will have false-negative result.

Most patients referred for suspected appendicitis will not have appendicitis. In fact, 50% of patients will have no aetiology found on examination for the pain, 25% will have appendicitis and the other 25% will have a variety of genito-urinary or gastrointestinal abnormalities.

COLOUR FLOW

Can be used to demonstrate colour flow through the periphery of the appendix reflecting hyperperfusion accompanying inflammation (Fig. 6.18).

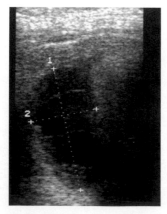

Figure 6.21 — Small pelvic collection post appendicectomy which appears cystic with septations.

Further reading

Abu-Yousef MM, Bleicher JJ, Maher JW, Urdaneta LF, Franken EA Jr, Metcalf AM. High-resolution sonography of acute appendicitis. *AJR* 1987; **149**: 53–58.

Agha FP, Ghahremani GG, Panella JS, Kaufman MW. Appendicitis as the initial manifestation of Crohn's disease: radiologic features and prognosis. *AJR* 1987; **149**: 515–518.

Alexander JE, Williamson SL, Seibert JJ, Golladay ES, Jimenez JF. The ultrasonographic diagnosis of typhlitis (neutropenic colitis). *Pediatr Radiol* 1988; **18**: 200–204.

Baker DE, Silver TM, Coran AG, McMillin KI. Postappendectomy fluid collections in children: incidence, nature, and evolution evaluated using US. *Radiology* 1986; **161**: 341–344.

Barr LL, Hayden CK Jr, Stansberry SD, Swischuk LE. Enteric duplication cysts in children: are their ultrasonographic wall characteristics diagnostic? *Pediatr Radiol* 1990; **20**: 326–328.

Biller JA, Grand RJ, Harris BH. Abdominal abscesses in adolescents with Crohn's disease. *J Pediatr Surg* 1987; **22(9)**: 873–876.

Bisset RAL, Gupta SC. Hypertrophic pyloric stenosis, ultrasonic appearances in a small baby. *Pediatr Radiol* 1988; **18**: 405.

Blumhagen JD, Noble HGS. Muscle thickness in hypertrophic pyloric stenosis: sonographic determination. *AJR* 1983; **140**: 221–223.

Borushok KF, Jeffrey RB Jr, Laing FC, Townsend PR. Sonographic diagnosis of perforation in patients with acute appendicitis. *AJR* 1990; **154**: 275–279.

Bowerman RA, Silver TM, Jaffe MH. Real-time ultrasound diagnosis of intussusception in children. *Radiology* 1982; **143**: 527–529.

Ceres L, Alonso I, Lopez P, Parra G, Echeverry J. Ultrasound study of acute appendicitis in children with emphasis upon the diagnosis of retrocecal appendicitis. *Pediatr Radiol* 1990; **20(4)**: 258–261.

Dinkel E, Dittrich M, Peters H, Baumann W. Real-time ultrasound in Crohn's disease: characteristic features and clinical implications. *Pediatr Radiol* 1986; **16**: 8–12.

Glasier CM, Siegel MJ, McAlister WH, Schackelford GD. Henoch-Schönlein syndrome in children: gastrointestinal manifestations. *AJR* 1981; **136**: 1081–1085.

Glass-Royal MC, Choyke PL, Gootenberg JE, Grant EG. Sonography in the diagnosis of neutropenic colitis. *J Ultrasound Med* 1987; **6**: 671–673.

Godbole P, Sprigg A, Dickson JA, Lin PC. Ultrasound compared with clinical examination in infantile hypertrophic pyloric stenosis. *Arch Dis Child* 1996; **75(4)**: 335–337.

Hadidi AT, El-Shal N. Childhood intussusception: a comparative study of nonsurgical management. *J Pediatr Surg* 1999; **34(2)**: 304–307.

Hahn HB, Hoepner FU, Kalle T, Macdonald EB, Prantl F, Spitzer IM, Faerber DR Sonography of acute appendicitis in children: 7 years experience. *Pediatr Radiol* 1998; **28(3)**: 147–151.

Haller JO, Cohen HL. Hypertrophic pyloric stenosis: diagnosis using US. *Radiology* 1986; **161**: 335–339.

Hayden CK Jr, Boulden TF, Swischuk LE, Lobe TE. Sonographic demonstration of duodenal obstruction with midgut volvulus. *AJR* 1984; **143**: 9–10.

Hayden CK Jr, Kuchelmeister J, Lipscomb TS. Sonography of acute appendicitis in childhood: perforation versus nonperforation. *J Ultrasound Med* 1992; **11**: 209–216.

Hu SC, Feeney MS, McNicholas M, O'Halpin D, Fitzgerald RJ. Ultrasonography to diagnose and exclude intussusception in Henoch-Schönlein purpura. *Arch Dis Child* 1991; **66(9)**: 1065–1067.

Kenney IJ. Ultrasound in intussusception: a false cystic lead point. *Pediatr Radiol* 1990; **20(5)**: 348.

Leonidas JC, Magid N, Soberman N, Glass TS. Midgut volvulus in infants: diagnosis with US. *Radiology* 1991; **179**: 491–493

Loyer E, Eggli KD. Sonographic evaluation of superior mesenteric vascular relationship in malrotation. *Pediatr Radiol* 1989; **19**: 173–175.

Macpherson RI. Gastrointestinal tract duplications: clinical, pathologic, etiologic, and radiologic considerations. *Radiographics* 1993; **13**: 1063–1080.

MacSweeney EJ, Oades PJ, Buchdahl R, Rosenthal M, Bush A. Relation of thickening of colon wall to pancreatic-enzyme treatment in cystic fibrosis. *Lancet* 1995; **25**; 345(8952): 752–756.

Martinez-Frontanilla LA, Silverman L, Meagher DP Jr. Intussusception in Henoch-Schönlein purpura: diagnosis with ultrasound. *J Pediatr Surg* 1988; **23**: 375–376.

McAlister WH, Kronemer KA. Emergency gastrointestinal radiology of the newborn. *Radiol Clin North Am* 1996; **34(4)**: 819–844.

Okorie NM, Dickson JAS, Carver RA, Steiner GM. What happens to the pylorus after pyloromyotomy? *Arch Dis Child* 1988; **63(11)**: 1339–1341.

Quillin SP, Siegel MJ, Coffin CM. Acute appendicitis in children: value of sonography in detecting perforation. *AJR* 1992; **159**: 1265–1268.

Quillin SP, Siegel MJ. Appendicitis: efficacy of color Doppler sonography. *Radiology* 1994; **191**: 557–560.

Quillin SP, Siegel MJ. Appendicitis in children: color Doppler sonography. *Radiology* 1992; **184**: 745–747.

Siegel MJ. *Pediatric Sonography.* 2nd ed. New York: Raven Press, 1995.

Smet MH, Marchal G, Ceulemans R, Eggermont E. The solitary hyperdynamic pulsating superior mesenteric artery: an additional dynamic sonographic feature of midgut volvulus. *Pediatr Radiol* 1991; **21**: 156–157.

Stringer MD, Capps SN, Pablot SM. Sonographic detection of the lead point in intussusception. *Arch Dis Child* 1992; **67(4)**: 529–530.

Zerin JM, DiPietro MA. Superior mesenteric vascular anatomy at US in patients with surgically proved malrotation of the mid-gut. *Radiology* 1992; **183**: 693–694.

7

THE
LIVER, GALLBLADDER,
BILIARY TREE

THE LIVER

Anatomy

The liver is located under the diaphragm in the right upper quadrant of the abdomen. It has three lobes: the right, left and caudate. The right lobe is the largest. The right and left lobes each have two segments, important surgically and distinguishable by ultrasound by the hepatic veins (Fig. 7.1).

The left lobe varies in size and can either be located entirely on the right side of the abdomen or can cross the midline to the left (Fig. 7.2).

The caudate lobe is usually located in the midline cephalad to the head of pancreas and anterior to the inferior vena cava (IVC) (Fig. 7.3). It is anatomically distinct because its blood supply is from both right and left hepatic arteries. Its portal vein and hepatic venous blood drains directly into the IVC.

In situs inversus the liver is located on the left side of the abdomen. Accessory lobes of the liver may occur on the inferior surface of the liver and are an incidental finding.

The most common accessory lobe is the Reidels lobe and is a caudal extension of the anterior margin of the right lobe which can often be mistaken clinically for a mass. It has a normal liver echotexture and merges imperceptibly with the normal right lobe.

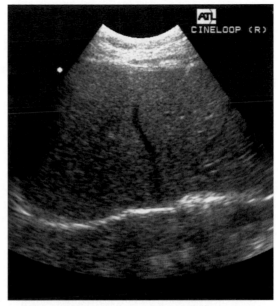

Figure 7.2 — Transverse section in the cephalic portion of the liver showing the left lobe to cross the midline to the left.

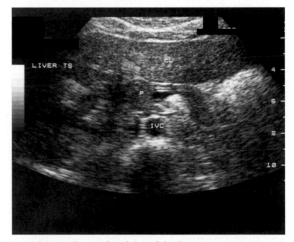

Figure 7.3 — The caudate lobe of the liver in transverse section cephalad to the head of pancreas (P) and anterior to the IVC.

Agenesis of the right or left lobe is a rare anomaly associated with volvulus, choledochal cyst and partial or complete absence of the right hemidiaphragm. There may be compensatory hypertrophy of other segments.

Portal veins

The portal vein carries blood from the spleen, mesentery and GI tract to the liver; 75% of the liver's blood volume is in the portal venous system. It is best

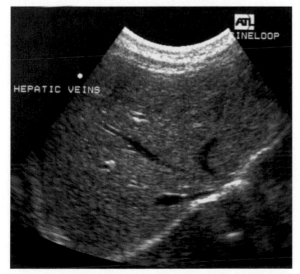

Figure 7.1 — Transverse section of the liver showing the hepatic veins; the middle hepatic vein divides the liver into the right and left lobes.

assessed in transverse sections as the larger branches course through the liver horizontally. The main portal vein is formed at the level of the pancreatic neck by the splenic and superior mesenteric vein and bifurcates at the porta hepatis into the right and left portal veins (Fig. 7.4).

The right portal vein continues transversely into the substance of the liver and divides into anterior and posterior branches supplying the anterior and posterior segments of the right lobe.

The left portal vein is of narrower calibre; it passes upwards and transversely through the left lobe of liver to the caudate lobe and then divides into the medial and lateral branches supplying the medial and lateral segments of the left lobe.

The left portal vein communicates with the obliterated umbilical vein which forms the ligamentum teres within the falciform ligament. In the newborn infant the patent umbilical vein may still be identified. The portal vein, at its junction with the umbilical vein, gives rise to the ductus venosus. The ductus venosus empties into the hepatic veins at their junction with the IVC.

Flow can be seen within the ductus venosus in all neonates in the first two days of life but persists in only 10% of neonates at 20 days. The ductus venosus may calcify once closed and may be identified as an echogenic linear focus with acoustic shadowing in the left lower lobe.

ULTRASOUND APPEARANCES

- The portal veins have an echogenic rim due to the fat tissue content of the walls of the vessels.

- Large calibre of the main portal vein at the porta hepatis is therefore easily recognised.

- Mean diameter of main portal vein: 8.5 ± 2.7 mm in patients less than 10 years of age; 10 ± 2 mm in patients 10–20 years.

- The portal veins within the liver are too small to be seen individually and appear as small round echogenic areas.

Hepatic veins

There are three major hepatic veins: the right, left and middle, which transport blood from the liver into the systemic circulation. They drain into the IVC (Fig. 7.5).

The right hepatic vein lies in the fissure between the anterior and posterior segments of the right lobe.

The middle hepatic vein lies in the fissure between the right and left lobes and in longitudinal section can be seen to drain into the IVC (Fig. 7.6).

The left hepatic vein lies in the fissure between the medial and lateral segments of the left lobe.

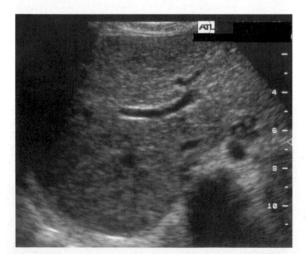

Figure 7.4 — Transverse section at a cephalad level showing the portal vein dividing into the right and left branches and the left subdividing into the medial and lateral branches.

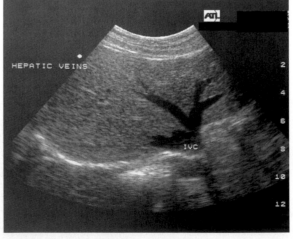

Figure 7.5 — Transverse section of the liver demonstrates the right, middle and left hepatic veins at their confluence with the IVC.

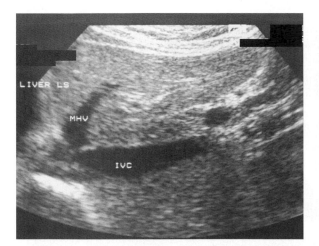

Figure 7.6 — Longitudinal section demonstrates the middle hepatic vein (MHV) draining into the IVC.

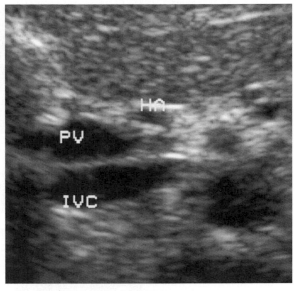

Figure 7.7 — Transverse section at the porta hepatis showing the location of the hepatic artery, anterior and medial to the main portal vein.

TECHNIQUE

Hepatic veins are best imaged in transverse section with the probe angled cephalad through the liver. They become larger in size as they approach their junction with the IVC.

Hepatic arteries

The arteries of the liver travel with the bile ducts and portal vein branches.

The normal sized intrahepatic arteries are not large enough to be imaged by ultrasound.

The common hepatic artery arises from the coeliac axis and crosses to the right superior anterior border of the pancreas to enter the porta hepatis.

At the porta hepatis the hepatic artery is located anteriorly and medially to the main portal vein (Fig. 7.7).

COLOUR FLOW DOPPLER AT THE PORTA HEPATIS

Colour flow Doppler is a useful technique for evaluating the hepatic vessels.

Portal vein (PV): displays low velocity, monophasic waveform (Fig. 7.8).

Hepatic vein (HV): multiphasic waveform with antegrade and retrograde flow reflecting changes with respiration (Fig. 7.9). The valsalva manoeuvre will reduce the HV pulsatility.

Hepatic artery (HA): characterised by high diastolic flow (Fig. 7.10).

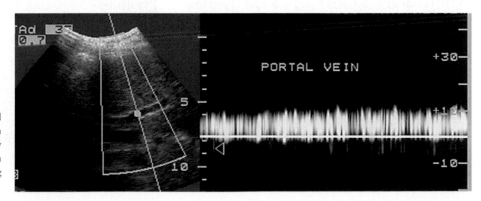

Figure 7.8 — Spectral Doppler of the portal vein demonstrating a low velocity monophasic waveform with slight increase of flow during inspiration.

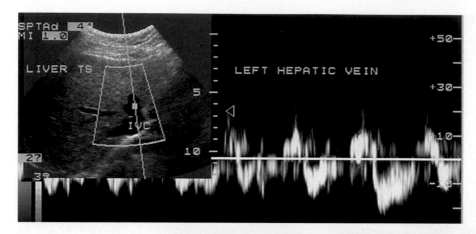

Figure 7.9 — Spectral Doppler waveform of the left hepatic vein displaying a multiphasic waveform.

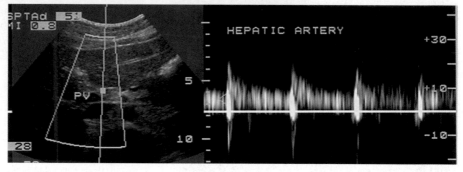

Figure 7.10 — Spectral Doppler waveform of the hepatic artery characterised by high diastolic flow.

Ligaments

The falciform ligament extends from the diaphragm to the umbilicus and contained within it is the ligamentum teres.

Ligamentum teres borders the medial and lateral segments of the left lobe.

Ligamentum venosum separates the caudate lobe and the lateral segment of the left lobe.

ULTRASOUND APPEARANCES

- Ligaments appear highly echogenic in comparison to the hepatic parenchyma because of the fatty tissue within and around them.

- Ligamentum teres, on longitudinal section, is seen as a hyperechoic line extending from the anterior surface of the liver to the left portal vein. On transverse section it is seen as a round hyperechoic area in the midline (Fig. 7.11).

- Ligamentum venosum is seen as a hyperechoic line anterior to the caudate lobe (Fig. 7.12).

ULTRASOUND APPEARANCES OF THE NORMAL LIVER

- The hepatic parenchyma has a fine homogeneous echotexture (Fig. 7.13).

- Within the parenchyma are small hyperechogenic round areas due to periportal fibrofatty tissue, highly echogenic linear structures caused by fissures and ligaments and fluid-filled vessels.

- In the neonate and up to 6 months of age the parenchyma of the liver is equally echogenic to that of the renal cortex (Fig. 7.14).

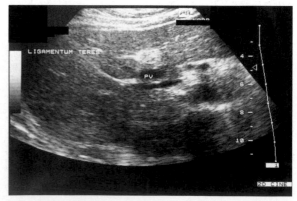

Figure 7.11 — Transverse section. The ligamentum teres appears as a round echogenic area in the midline.

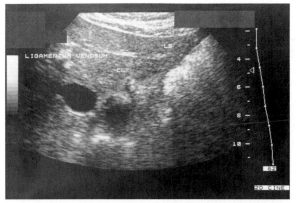

Figure 7.12 — Transverse section. The ligamentum venosum appears as an echogenic line anterior to the caudate lobe (CL). It separates the caudate lobe and the lateral segment (LS) of the left lobe.

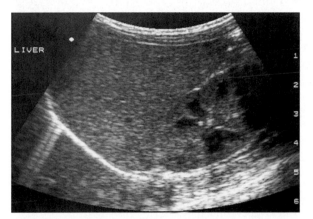

Figure 7.13 — Longitudinal section of the normal liver displaying a fine homogeneous echotexture.

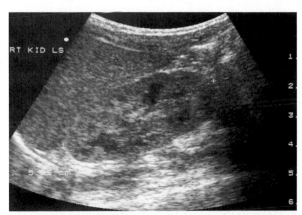

Figure 7.14 — In the neonate and up to 6 months of age normal echogenicity of the liver is equal to that of the renal cortex (2-month-old male).

- After 6 months of age the liver is usually more echogenic than the kidney (Fig. 7.15).
- The liver is slightly hypoechoic in comparison with the spleen.

CHOICE OF TRANSDUCER

3.5 MHz curved for older children as this affords greater penetration.

5 MHz curved in neonates – and up to approximately 10 years.

PATIENT PREPARATION

For the liver alone no preparation is required. If the gallbladder is also to be imaged, ideally the patient should be fasted for 4–6 hours before ultrasound examination, to ensure adequate distension of the gallbladder. It is always worth attempting a non-fasting examination as adequate information may be obtained.

TECHNIQUE

The patient is examined in the supine and left posterior oblique position using either a 3.5 or 5.0 MHz curved transducer. The depth of the image should be adjusted to include the posterior surface of the liver. Further adjustments to the output, gain and time gain compensation controls should be made so that the parenchyma of the liver appears homogeneous from the anterior to the posterior surface.

In children the liver can be imaged using a subcostal approach. Longitudinal, transverse sections and standard views should be obtained so that the liver is imaged systematically.

All parts of the liver, hepatic and portal veins, common hepatic artery, bile duct and gallbladder fossa should be examined.

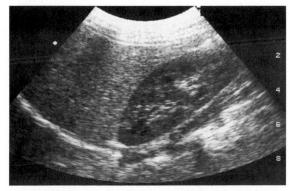

Figure 7.15 — After 6 months of age normal echogenicity of the liver is more echogenic than kidney (8-year-old female).

Hepatomegaly

Definition : enlargement of the liver so that it is clinically palpable (Fig. 7.16).

CAUSES

Masses:

1° tumours: (malignant)	Hepatoblastoma Hepatic carcinoma Hepatoma	

2° tumour: Metastases Lymphoma

1° tumours: (benign)   Hepatic cysts
Haemangioma
Haemangioendothelioma
Hamartoma
Adenoma
Focal nodular hyperplasia

Cardiac failure

Metabolic diseases, e.g. glycogen storage disease

Infection, e.g. hepatitis, hepatic abscess

Cirrhosis, e.g. biliary atresia, cystic fibrosis

Syndromes: with organomegaly, e.g. Beckwith's syndrome.

ULTRASOUND APPEARANCES

Appearance varies with cause of hepatomegaly:

- Discrete lesions, e.g. tumours, are hypo or hyperechoic.

- Diffuse disease
  - even increase in echotexture
  - even decrease in echotexture
  - mixed attenuation with loss of normal appearance.

Liver cysts

These are rare in children and are congenital or acquired, single or multiple.

Congenital: solitary and usually located in the inferior portion of the right lobe. May be identified antenatally. Must be distinguished from choledochal cysts.

Multiple cysts: Autosomal dominant polycystic disease, Van Hippel-Lindau disease.

Mesenchymal hamartoma of the liver.

Acquired: echinococcal disease, abscess (amoebic in endemic areas), evolving haematomas.

CLINICAL PRESENTATION

Abdominal mass.

Pain, hepatomegaly, jaundice.

ULTRASOUND APPEARANCES

Congenital

- Anechoic, well-defined lesions.
- Round or oval in shape with thin walls (Fig. 7.17a,b).
- Variable degrees of acoustic enhancement.
- Usually unilocular but occasionally internal septations can be seen.

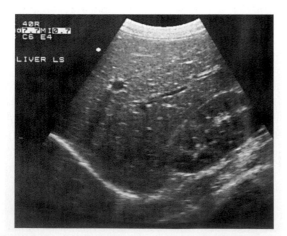

Figure 7.16 — Longitudinal section illustrating hepatomegaly of the liver; the right lobe overhangs the upper pole of the right kidney.

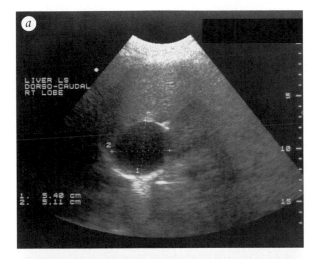

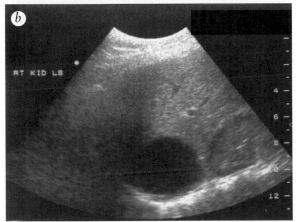

Figure 7.17 — Single, anechoic cyst within the RLL: (a) well-defined, thin-walled with posterior acoustic enhancement and (b) separate from the right kidney.

Acquired

Abscess (amoebic) and resolving haematomas can at times appear anechoic with well-defined walls.

Echinococcal typically hypoechoic lesion with internal echoes due to debris. Can have daughter cysts. Some can be anechoic and resemble congenital cysts.

TREATMENT

Percutaneous needle aspiration may be required for diagnosis.

Percutaneous drainage of an abscess.

Surgical excision, sclerosis or internal drainage may be required.

MERITS

Ultrasound is 95–100% accurate in diagnosing hepatic cysts.

LIMITATIONS

If the cyst is pedunculated and the area of attachment to the liver is not identified, then the origin of the mass may be incorrectly assigned to the mesentery, omentum or ovary. CT/MR may be needed for further evaluation.

ASSOCIATED ANOMALIES

Autosomal dominant polycystic disease.

Von Hippel-Lindau disease.

Abscess

Definition: The result of bacterial spread from organisms such as *Escherichia coli* and *Staphylococcus aureus*.

Can occur in any part of the liver although approximately 80% are located in the posterior portion of the right lobe.

CLINICAL PRESENTATION

Upper abdominal pain and/or tenderness.

Fever.

Hepatomegaly.

Raised liver function tests (LFT's).

ULTRASOUND APPEARANCES

• Variable in appearance with a broad spectrum of echogenicity ranging from anechoic to highly echogenic (Fig. 7.18).

• Irregular, variable in size, septations.

• Thick walled, debris and fluid levels.

TREATMENT

Percutaneous needle aspiration for diagnosis.

Drainage, usually percutaneous.

Antibiotic therapy.

Trauma

Mostly blunt abdominal trauma, includes hepatic laceration, fractures, haematoma and haemoperitoneum; also stab wounds and lacerations.

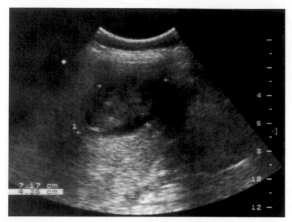

Figure 7.18 — Liver abscess within the right lobe. Variable echogenicity due to debris and fluid. Irregular in outline.

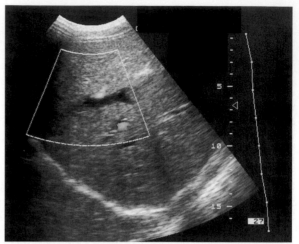

Figure 7.19 — Trauma: hepatic laceration within RLL shown as a linear defect of the parenchyma with no blood flow demonstrated on colour flow imaging.

CLINICAL PRESENTATION

Acute abdomen.

ULTRASOUND APPEARANCES

- Hepatic lacerations appear as linear or branching defects of the liver parenchyma (Fig. 7.19). May have associated subcapsular collection.

- Hepatic fractures have linear defect traversing the entire lobe or segment.
  May have associated subcapsular collection.

- Hepatic haematomas show a focal collection of blood, oval or round with smooth or irregular margins.

- Subcapsular collections will flatten the lateral aspect of the liver.

- Vary in appearance with age of the haematoma.

  If acute: appear hyperechoic due to the presence of blood clot.

  After 2–3 days: appear hypoechoic and cystic as blood liquefies.

- Haemoperitoneum are variable in size and may be located in the right subphrenic and subhepatic spaces or if larger can be found in the paracolic gutter and pelvic cul-de-sac.

TREATMENT

Mostly conservative management.

Most intrahepatic injuries resolve spontaneously within weeks to months.

Surgical intervention, if required, is based on clinical assessment and not the imaging findings.

LIMITATIONS

CT is the preferred method of determining the presence and extent of liver trauma. Once hepatic injury has been established, ultrasonography is indicated to monitor progress.

Cirrhosis

This causes chronic destruction of hepatic parenchyma which is replaced by fibrosis and nodular regeneration.

Causes of cirrhosis in childhood include: cystic fibrosis, biliary atresia, chronic hepatitis and metabolic diseases.

ULTRASOUND APPEARANCES

- Coarse parenchyma with increased echogenicity (Fig. 7.20).

- Nodular margins to the liver.

- Initial liver enlargement, then the liver may become small.

- Small right lobe of liver.

- Hypertrophy of the left and caudate lobes.

- Secondary signs of cirrhosis include ascites, splenomegaly and varices associated with portal hypertension.

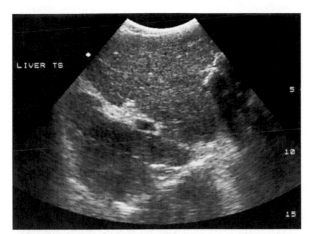

Figure 7.20 — Cirrhotic liver associated with cystic fibrosis. Note coarse liver parenchyma with fibrotic changes.

Once cirrhosis is detected, the examination should always include Doppler studies of the portal vein to look for reverse flow indicating portal hypertension.

Malignant liver tumours

Third most common neoplasm in children after Wilms' and neuroblastoma. Usually hepatoblastomas or hepatocellular carcinomas.

CLINICAL PRESENTATION

Upper abdominal mass.

Abdominal fullness/pain.

Raised LFT's.

Weight loss.

Fever.

Diarrhoea and vomiting.

Hepatoblastoma, more common in children under 5 years of age, usually occurs in isolation. There is a known association with Beckwith-Weidemann syndrome. Hepatocellular carcinoma is more common in children over 5 years of age.

ULTRASOUND APPEARANCES
- Similar ultrasound appearances to hepatoblastoma and hepatocellular carcinoma.
- Usually confined to one lobe (usually right lobe).

- Appear most frequently as solitary masses, or a dominant mass with smaller lesions.
- Rarer are multiple nodules throughout the liver.
- Most tumours are hyperechoic and heterogeneous due to necrosis and haemorrhage (Fig. 7.21).
- Calcification: echogenic foci with acoustic shadowing (Fig. 7.22). More frequent in hepatoblastoma.
- Diffuse involvement is rare: heterogeneous parenchyma with distorted vascular architecture.
- The examination must include colour Doppler studies.
- Intravascular infiltration: echogenic thrombus within lumen of vessel, e.g. portal or hepatic veins.
- On colour flow imaging: blood flow within or around tumour can be observed.

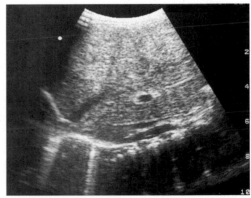

Figure 7.21 — Hepatoblastoma of the right lobe in 2-year-old male; abnormal liver texture due to necrosis and haemorrhage.

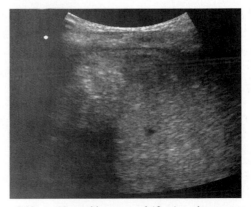

Figure 7.22 — Hepatoblastoma calcification demonstrated as echogenic foci with acoustic shadowing.

TREATMENT

Chemotherapy followed by surgical resection.

LIMITATIONS

Definitive diagnosis requires tissue sampling. Caution is needed with percutaneous biopsy because these lesions are highly vascular.

MR for further evaluation of the tumour to define extent and suitability for surgery.

CT of the chest for metastases.

Cavernous haemangioma

Benign hepatic tumours of vascular origin containing multiple dilated blood-filled spaces.

Lined with endothelial cells and separated by fibrous septa.

Typically affect older children and adolescents.

Majority are located in the posterior segment of the right lobe.

CLINICAL PRESENTATION

Asymptomatic, usually incidental finding.

Occasionally a child presents with enlarged abdomen or hepatomegaly.

ULTRASOUND APPEARANCES

- Round, homogeneous hyperechoic lesions with well-defined margins (Fig. 7.23).

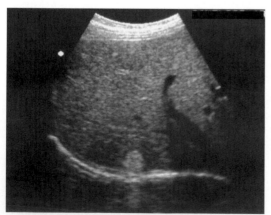

Figure 7.23 — Benign cavernous haemangioma. Round, homogeneous, hyperechoic 1.5 cm lesion with well defined margins in the right lobe of the liver (note mirror artefact at diaphragm).

- Usually less than 3 cm in diameter.

- Become heterogeneous or hypoechoic as they undergo degeneration, thrombosis and fibrosis. This process begins at the centre of the lesion, therefore can have a hyperechoic mass with a hypoechoic centre.

- Posterior enhancement is seen in over 75%.

- Slow blood flow within the lesion on colour flow imaging.

LIMITATIONS

Sonographic finding of cavernous haemangioma can be non-specific and further imaging is required, e.g. CT, MR, scintigraphy to reach a definitive diagnosis.

Congenital haemangioma / haemangioendotheliomas

Benign tumour of vascular origin.

Present in the neonatal period.

Often with cardiac failure.

Hepatomegaly.

ULTRASOUND APPEARANCES

- Right lobe of liver but may affect both.

- Echoic appearances depends on necrosis; usually echogenic margins with hypoechoic centre.

- Usually solitary but may be multiple, especially haemangioendotheliomas and in Kasabach Merritt syndrome.

- Acoustic enhancement.

- Colour flow studies show hypervascularity.

- Needs further cross sectional imaging.

TREATMENT

May need embolisation.

Mesenchymal hamartoma

A rare, benign tumour with multiple cysts, found in children under 2 years of age with boys affected twice as often as girls.

CLINICAL PRESENTATION

Asymptomatic abdominal mass.

Congestive heart failure.

ULTRASOUND APPEARANCES

- Well circumscribed, multilocular masses containing anechoic spaces separated by echogenic septa (Fig. 7.24). If bleeding occurs the cysts became echogenic.

- Can look like autosomal dominant polycystic disease but the kidneys are normal.

OTHER PROCEDURES

Cross sectional imaging by MR to evaluate fully.

TREATMENT

Surgical resection.

Liver adenoma

A benign lesion composed entirely of hepatocytes, associated with glycogen storage disease.

CLINICAL PRESENTATION

Hepatomegaly.

Abdominal enlargement.

ULTRASOUND APPEARANCES

- Solitary, well circumscribed (Fig. 7.25).

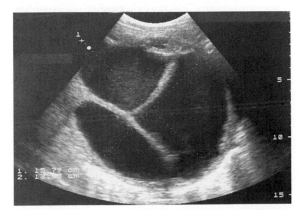

Figure 7.24 — Mesenchymal hamartoma of the liver in a 2-year-old male. A well-circumscribed, multilocular mass containing anechoic spaces separated by echogenic septa is demonstrated.

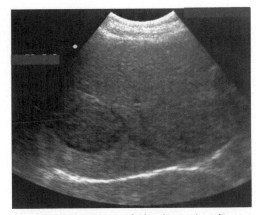

Figure 7.25 — Adenoma of the liver. A solitary, well-circumscribed benign lesion in the RLL.

- Vary from isoechoic to hypoechoic.

- If bleeding has occurred may be hyperechoic or mixed echoes.

Focal nodular hyperplasia

A benign lesion of the liver composed of an abnormal arrangement of normal hepatocytes, Kupffer cells and bile ducts.

CLINICAL PRESENTATION

Hepatomegaly.

ULTRASOUND APPEARANCES

- Usually a solitary lesion, slightly hypoechoic to normal parenchyma. May demonstrate echogenic centre (Fig. 7.26a–c).

- Detected due to mass effect on adjacent vessels.

Metastases

Tumours that metastasise to the liver include:

Rhabdoid Wilms' tumour

Stage IV neuroblastoma

Rhabdomyosarcoma

Lymphoma

Sacrococcygeal teratoma

Hepatic tumours.

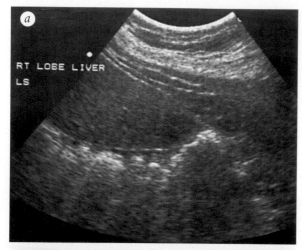

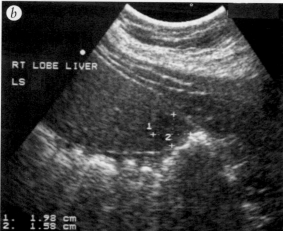

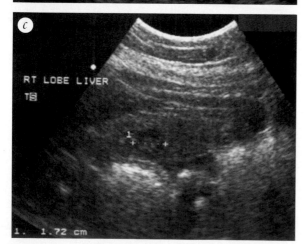

Figure 7.26 — Focal nodular hyperplasia. Solitary lesion in the right lobe of liver: slightly hypoechoic to surrounding normal liver parenchyma in longitudinal section (a & b) and with an echogenic centre in transverse section (c).

ULTRASOUND APPEARANCES

- Solitary or multiple hypoechoic lesions in either lobe (Fig. 7.27).

- Variable size.

- Usually found during routine screening.

Liver transplant

Preoperative evaluation

To determine patency of the extrahepatic portal vein as any narrowing or occlusion makes surgical anastomosis difficult or impossible.

Normal antegrade flow should be demonstrated in the extrahepatic portal vein.

If portal flow is absent or diminished or collaterals are present, then angiography or MRI is required for further vascular assessment.

The IVC, hepatic artery and veins should also be evaluated for patency. The suprahepatic portion of the IVC must be patent for transplantation.

Postoperative evaluation

To determine patency of the hepatic artery as thrombosis of the hepatic artery is the most common vascular complication of liver transplantation.

If the hepatic artery is thrombosed there will be absence of hepatic arterial waveform in the porta, both lobes of

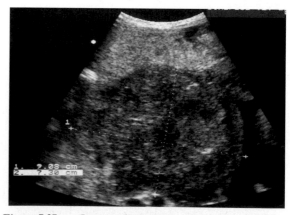

Figure 7.27 — Large, solitary lesion of mixed echogenicity measuring 9 × 7 cm within the right lobe of the liver (metastases of rhabdomyosarcoma).

liver and region of anastomosis. There will be decreased diastolic flow and increased resistive indices.

False-negative and false-positive diagnoses of hepatic artery thrombosis can be made and if clinically suspected MRI or angiography should be performed.

Portal vein thrombosis and stenosis are also complications.

Other complications include: fluid collections, biliary obstruction, abnormal liver texture secondary to rejection, infection, abscess, arteriovenous fistulas.

Viral hepatitis

Infection of the liver.

Type A is most frequent in children.

B, C occur in AIDS, drug abusers, or in patients treated with contaminated IV blood products.

CLINICAL PRESENTATION
Jaundice with dark urine and pale stools.

RUQ pain.

Lethargy and fever – variable.

ULTRASOUND APPEARANCES
● Liver is usually normal.

In acute hepatitis

● Hepatomegaly.
● Diffuse hypoechoic parenchyma with increased periportal echogenicity (Fig. 7.28).

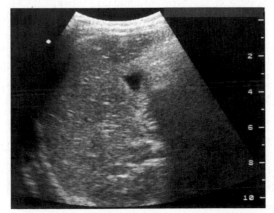

Figure 7.28 — Transverse section showing a diffusely hypoechoic liver with periportal echogenicity consistent with acute hepatitis.

● Thick-walled gallbladder.
● Enlarged lymph nodes.

In chronic hepatitis

● Increased echogenicity of parenchyma becoming heterogeneous.
● Small gallbladder with sludge or stones.

Neonatal hepatitis

A common cause of neonatal cholestasis and thought to be due to infection antenatally resulting from injury to hepatocytes.

AGE RANGE
3–4 weeks of age.

CLINICAL PRESENTATION
Obstructive jaundice.

ULTRASOUND APPEARANCES
● Similar to those found in biliary atresia.
● Hepatic echogenicity can be normal, increased or heterogeneous, depending on the degree of cirrhosis.
● Normal calibre of intra- and extrahepatic bile ducts.
● The gallbladder can be large, normal, small or not visualised.
● The finding of an enlarged or normal gallbladder favours a diagnosis of neonatal hepatitis.
● The gallbladder will change size with feeding in patients with neonatal hepatitis.

OTHER PROCEDURES
Radionuclide imaging (Tc^{99}m HIDA).

TREATMENT
Managed medically.

Fatty infiltration of the liver

Can be diffuse or focal.

Associated with cystic fibrosis.

Occurs with malnutrition.

May occur with severe debilitation.

Alcoholism (in adults).

CLINICAL PRESENTATION

Usually incidental finding of enlarged liver and deranged liver function tests when investigating failure to thrive.

ULTRASOUND APPEARANCES

- Echobright liver with diffuse infiltration (Fig. 7.29).
- Hepatomegaly.

Portal hypertension

In childhood, this is most commonly due to portal vein thrombosis.

It also occurs with cirrhosis.

CLINICAL PRESENTATION

Variable.

Enlarged spleen.

Haematemesis due to variceal bleeding.

ULTRASOUND APPEARANCES

- Enlarged spleen.
- Absent flow in the portal vein if thrombosed.

- Reverse flow on Doppler ultrasound in splenic vein.
- Collateral veins replacing the normal portal vein.
- Cavernoma: multiple tortuous vessels in the porta due to collaterals (Fig. 7.30).
- Occasionally see varices at the distal oesophagus.
- May see reopening of ductus venosum.

TREATMENT

Medical management.

Portocaval shunt by TIPS.

Liver transplant.

Sclerotherapy of varices.

THE GALLBLADDER

Anatomy

Elliptical structure located in a fossa between the right and left lobes of the undersurface of the liver.

The gallbladder has 3 parts: fundus, body and neck.

The caudal portion is oval which narrows down to a tubular structure as it joins the cystic duct.

Folds can occur in the gallbladder; the most common are the phrygian cap (Fig. 7.31a), which is a fold in the

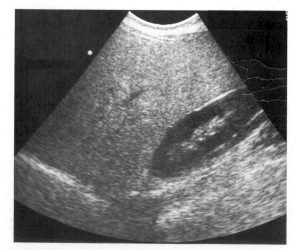

Figure 7.29 — Diffuse fatty infiltration in a 12-year-old girl with cystic fibrosis, demonstrating hepatomegaly with increased echogenicity of the liver compared to the kidney.

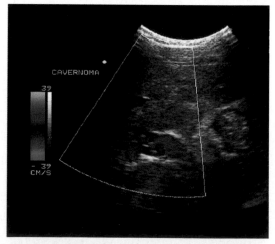

Figure 7.30 — Abnormal tortuous vessels of the portal vein at porta hepatis due to cavernomatous transformation secondary to portal vein thrombosis.

distal portion of the fundus, and the incisura (Fig. 7.31b), which is a fold between the body and the neck. Care must be taken to ensure that such folds are not mistaken for calculi or septae (Fig. 7.31c).

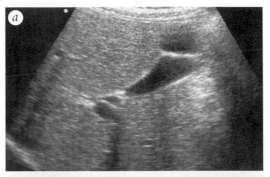

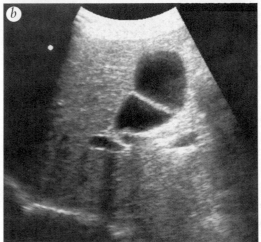

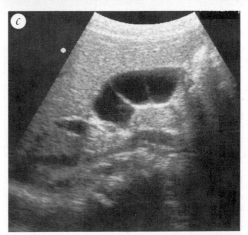

Figure 7.31 — Folds of the gallbladder: the phrygian cap (a) and the incisura fold (b) which should not be mistaken for septae within the gallbladder (c).

The gallbladder can lie in an ectopic position, e.g. between the liver and the diaphragm, below the left lobe of liver, or intrahepatically within the interlobar fissure but this is rare. Anatomical variations include duplication and multiseptate gallbladder – both very rare. The size of the gallbladder increases with patient age.

Infants up to 1 year: gallbladder length 1.5–3 cm.

Older children: gallbladder length 3–7 cm.

The size of the gallbladder varies depending on whether the patient has fasted or not.

A larger gallbladder after fasting with a round shape could suggest hydrops.

The normal distended gallbladder has a smooth wall with a thickness of 3 mm or less.

CHOICE OF TRANSDUCER
Curved 5 or 7/4 MHz.

For older children use curved 3.5 MHz.

PATIENT PREPARATION
Usually fasted for 4+ hours but always worth trying between meals. If you see it and it is normal, the child does not need a fasting study.

ULTRASOUND APPEARANCES
• The gallbladder appears as a sonolucent structure in the right upper quadrant.

• In longitudinal section it appears pear-shaped and in transverse section circular (Fig. 7.32a,b).

TECHNIQUE
Initially the patient is examined in the supine position. The transducer is placed midline in sagittal section on the patient's anterior abdominal wall at the level of the xiphisternum. The transducer is moved subcostally, using a continuous scanning action, towards the patient's right lower costal margin until the gallbladder is located. The patient may be repositioned from a supine position to a left posterior oblique position (rotated approximately 45 degrees to the patient's left) in order to help visualisation of the gallbladder.

Once located, the transducer is angled medially to laterally in an arcuate fashion to image the entire gallbladder in sagittal section. The transducer is then rotated

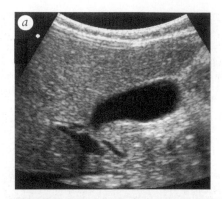

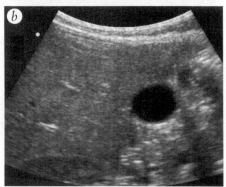

Figure 7.32 — Normal appearance of the gallbladder: (a) pear-shaped in longitudinal section and (b) circular in transverse section.

through 90 degrees over the gallbladder and multiple cranio-caudal movements of the transducer are made to image the entire gallbladder in transverse section. (Technique of measuring the common bile duct is included under Biliary Tree).

Sludge

Biliary sludge is viscous bile with particulate matter of calcium bilirubinate granules due to stasis of bile. Sludge is often the initial step in the development of gallstones.

CLINICAL PRESENTATION

Right upper quadrant pain ± fluctuating jaundice.

TECHNIQUE

Change of patient position (LPO or upright/erect) will demonstrate movement of sludge into the dependent part of the lumen.

ULTRASOUND APPEARANCES

- Low to medium level echoes without acoustic shadows (Fig. 7.33).

- Sludge moves slowly with change in patient position and layers in the dependent part of the lumen of the gallbladder.

- Sludge may form mobile masses called sludge balls or tumefactive sludge which appear echogenic but do not display acoustic shadowing (Fig. 7.34). They disappear spontaneously.

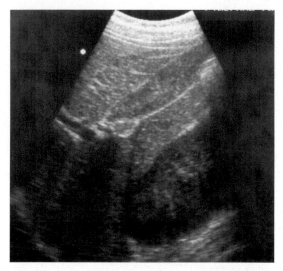

Figure 7.33 — Sludge. Low to medium level echoes filling the gallbladder without acoustic shadowing.

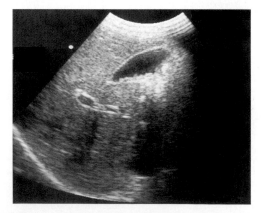

Figure 7.34 — Sludge within the gallbladder; echogenic material which does not display acoustic shadowing.

TREATMENT

This depends on underlying cause. Either none or occasionally surgical investigation.

LIMITATIONS

Care should be taken to avoid saturation of the image as misdiagnosis of sludge is possible.

Blood and pus, both very rare, may cause similar ultrasonic appearances.

Hydrops

A rare disorder with acute distension of the gallbladder without any obstruction.

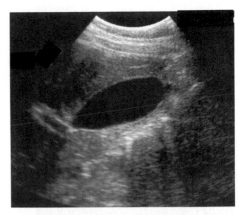

Figure 7.35 — Hydrops of the gallbladder in a patient with Kawasaki's disease. The longitudinal section demonstrates a biconvex appearance.

ASSOCIATION

Infection.

Kawasaki disease.

Polyarteritis nodosa.

Leptospirosis.

CLINICAL PRESENTATION

May be asymptomatic.

RUQ pain, vomiting ± mild jaundice.

Afebrile.

ULTRASOUND APPEARANCES

- No dilatation of the bile ducts.
- The bile is anechoic.
- The gallbladder is markedly distended (Fig. 7.35).

TREATMENT

Antibiotics and treatment of underlying disease. Usually resolves spontaneously.

Gallstones (Cholelithiasis)

Approximately 85% of children with gallstones have underlying diseases predisposing to stone formation.

In the remaining 15% stone formation is idiopathic.

Neonates undergoing parenteral nutrition, furosemide therapy and phototherapy are at risk of stone formation.

Up to 40% of infants receiving total parenteral nutrition develop stones due to bile stasis.

Causes of gallstones in older children include cystic fibrosis, total parenteral nutrition, Crohn's disease, malabsorption, congenital spherocytosis and congenital bile duct malformation.

CLINICAL PRESENTATION

Abdominal pain, usually intermittent rather than acute colic.

Jaundice which may fluctuate with passage of stones into the CBD.

Persistent jaundice if complete common bile duct obstruction.

Often incidental finding on routine surveillance in children at risk.

TECHNIQUE

A change in patient position may be required to eliminate false results.

ULTRASOUND APPEARANCES

- Echogenic foci with strong posterior acoustic shadowing (Fig. 7.36a) Rarely they can be non-shadowing.
- They are mobile and normally layer in the dependent part of the gallbladder lumen (Fig. 7.36b) but may float.

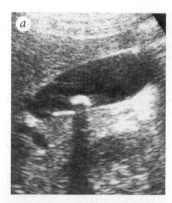

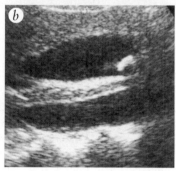

Figure 7.36 — Longitudinal section of the gallbladder showing (a) a single gallstone as an echogenic focus displaying a strong posterior acoustic shadow, and (b) the mobile gallstone which moves with a change in patient position.

- Acoustic shadowing is dependent on the position and size of the stone within the beam of ultrasound.

- Shadowing does not relate to the calcium content of the stone.

- The smaller the stone the more difficult it is to demonstrate acoustic shadowing.

TREATMENT

Depends on the underlying cause and may include no treatment, stone removal, leaving the gallbladder in situ, or cholecystectomy.

MERITS

Sensitivity for detecting gallstones is greater than 95%.

LIMITATIONS

False-negative diagnosis of gallstones is rare but can occur if:

The stone is impacted in the neck of the gallbladder or cystic duct.

The gallbladder is packed with stones and is mistaken for air-filled bowel due to the massive shadowing.

False positives can occur due to:

Shadowing in the region of the cystic duct which may result from the spiral valves of Heister and not from a stone.

Air-filled bowel with its associated shadowing can be mistaken for a stone-filled gallbladder.

Examination of the patient in varying positions will eliminate false-positive/negative result.

Differential diagnosis between a gallstone and polyp can be made by repositioning the patient. A polyp will not alter with patient position.

Cholecystitis

Acute

Inflammation of the gallbladder as a result of cystic duct obstruction secondary to calculi or by viscous bile due to stasis associated with recent surgery, sepsis, burns.

CLINICAL PRESENTATION

RUQ pain.

Fever.

Leukocytosis with or without jaundice.

TECHNIQUE

Include measurement of the gallbladder wall.

ULTRASOUND APPEARANCES

- Enlarged gallbladder.

- Gallbladder wall thickness greater than 3mm (seen in 50–75% of patients).

- Localised tenderness (Murphy's sign) on scanning.

- Sludge or gallstones may be present.

- Sonolucent rim/halo around thickened gallbladder wall representing oedema (Fig. 7.37).

Chronic

Inflammation of the gallbladder secondary to gallstones or CF.

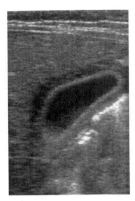

Figure 7.37 — Cholecystitis. Sonolucent rim/halo around thickened gallbladder wall representing oedema due to inflammation.

CLINICAL PRESENTATION

Chronic recurrent right upper quadrant pain.

ULTRASOUND APPEARANCES

- May be normal.
- Sludge.
- Gallstones.
- Thickened gallbladder wall.

Strawberry gallbladder adenomyomatosis

A variant of chronic cholecystitis which rarely occurs in childhood.

- Thickening of the wall with irregularity of the mucosal lining which may resemble small stones if this is localised.
- No alteration of appearances with position.
- The wall irregularity is due to prominence of the Rokitansky Aschoff sinuses.

BILIARY TREE

Anatomy

Bile enters bile capillaries that empty into small bile ducts which merge to form the larger right and left hepatic ducts. These unite to leave the liver as the common hepatic duct. The common bile duct is formed by the junction of the common hepatic duct and cystic ducts. The distal aspect of the common bile duct, after leaving the hepatoduodenal ligament, takes a downward and posterior course to enter the substance of the head of the pancreas. It then merges with the pancreatic duct to enter the duodenum at the ampulla.

CHOICE OF TRANSDUCER

Curved 5 MHz or 3.5 MHz for older children.

PATIENT PREPARATION

As for gallbladder examination.

TECHNIQUE

As for liver and gallbladder.

BILE DUCT MEASUREMENT

The patient is positioned in a left posterior oblique position and the transducer is placed in longitudinal section to image the extrahepatic portions of the biliary tree. Either the common hepatic duct or the common bile duct can be measured. Measurement of the bile duct should be made from internal to internal wall (Fig. 7.38a,b).

ULTRASOUND APPEARANCES

- Normally only a small segment of the extrahepatic biliary tree can be seen sonographically.
- The common hepatic duct can be identified anterior to the portal vein at the porta hepatis and the distal segment of the common bile duct can be identified anterior to the portal vein as it enters the head of pancreas.
- The bile ducts are anechoic and are seen in longitudinal section as tubular structures and in transverse section as rounded structures.
- The walls of the bile ducts are echogenic.
- Normally the CHD/CBD should not exceed 2 mm in diameter in infants under 1 year of age, 4 mm in older children and 7 mm in adolescents.

Obstruction

Dilated intra- or extrahepatic bile ducts.

The ducts dilate proximal to the site of obstruction.

Biliary obstruction can occur at 3 sites: the porta hepatis, suprapancreatic common duct, infrapancreatic common duct.

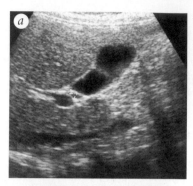

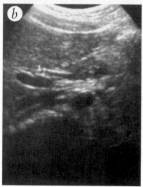

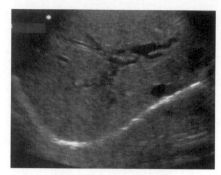

Figure 7.39 — Stellate branching appearance of dilated intrahepatic bile ducts which are seen as tubular, anechoic structures within the liver.

Figure 7.38 — (a) The common hepatic duct in a 10-year-old, seen anterior to the portal vein, is measured from internal to internal wall. (b) The distal segment of the common bile duct in a 13-year-old seen anterior to the portal vein at the level of the pancreas.

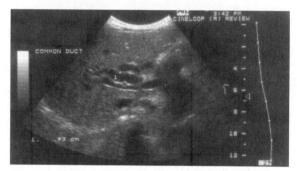

Figure 7.40 — Dilated common bile duct (9 mm calibre in 5½-year-old) seen anterior to portal vein.

CLINICAL PRESENTATION

May be symptomless.

Biliary colic.

Jaundice which may be intermittent.

Mass.

Pain.

Fever.

ULTRASOUND APPEARANCES

- Tubular anechoic structures within the liver.
- May have a stellate branching appearance (Fig. 7.39).
- Acoustic enhancement.
- Dilated common hepatic duct is seen anterior to right portal vein.
- Dilated CBD seen anterior to main portal vein (Fig. 7.40).

- Calculi can be present.
- 1° and 2° neoplasm: hypoechoic mass around the CBD or in region of porta hepatis and marked biliary tract dilatation.

OTHER PROCEDURES

Percutaneous cholangiography.

CT.

Radionuclide imaging.

MERITS

Colour flow imaging can be used to differentiate between dilated bile ducts and blood vessels.

Choledochal cyst

Congenital dilatation of the biliary ductal system.

Cause of choledochal cyst is unknown.

There are 3 types:

Type 1: dilatation of CBD.

Type 2: an eccentric diverticulum of the CBD.

Type 3: dilatation of the duodenal portion of the CBD (choledochocele).

Approximately 22% of patients present before 12 months of age, 33% between 1 and 10 years of age and 45% after 10 years of age.

CLINICAL PRESENTATION
Jaundice.

Abdominal pain.

Mass.

ULTRASOUND APPEARANCES
- A well-defined, fluid-filled mass separate from the gallbladder (Fig. 7.41a,b).

- Located in or near the porta hepatis.

- Dilatation of the intrahepatic bile ducts usually seen without proximal dilatation which helps to distinguish this from other causes of obstructive jaundice.

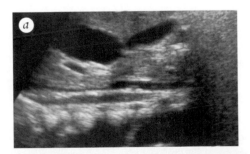

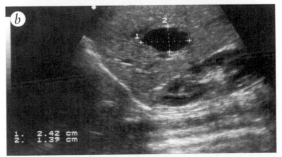

Figure 7.41 — Choledochal cyst (a & b) a well-defined, fluid-filled mass separate from the gallbladder.

TREATMENT
Surgery.

MERITS
Ultrasound in many instances can provide diagnosis.

Caroli's disease

Rare condition.

Congenital saccular dilatation of the major intrahepatic bile ducts without evidence of proximal obstruction.

Stone formation and cholangitis may occur.

Can be seen with congenital hepatic fibrosis and/or autosomal recessive polycystic kidney disease.

CLINICAL PRESENTATION
Pain.

Fever.

Jaundice.

ULTRASOUND APPEARANCES
- Multiple, dilated, tubular structures represent segmental dilatation of the intrahepatic bile ducts.

- Irregularity of the walls with nodular protrusions.

- Echogenic bands across the dilated bile duct lumina.

- Portal veins/radicles partially or completely surrounded by the dilated bile ducts.

- Intraluminal calculi.

OTHER PROCEDURES
Hepatobiliary scintigraphy.

MR cholangiography.

Biliary atresia

Common cause of neonatal cholestasis.

Thought to be a result of infection antenatally of the bile ducts in which part or all of the larger bile ducts can be obliterated.

AGE RANGE
3–4 weeks of age.

CLINICAL PRESENTATION

Obstructive jaundice.

ULTRASOUND APPEARANCES

- Intra- and extrahepatic bile ducts are normal in calibre. Hepatic echogenicity can be normal or increased depending on secondary cirrhosis.

- Gallbladder is usually small or not seen although in 10% of patients the gallbladder can appear normal.

- If seen it does not change with feeding.

- A rarer appearance is the finding of a solitary cyst in the biliary tree.

OTHER PROCEDURES

Radionuclide imaging (Tc^{99}m HIDA) is required to differentiate between biliary atresia and neonatal hepatitis.

ASSOCIATED ANOMALIES

Choledochal cyst.

Hydronephrosis.

Situs inversus.

Diaphragmatic hernia.

TREATMENT

Biliary atresia requires early surgical intervention with porto jejunostomy to prevent biliary cirrhosis – the Kasai procedure. The earlier the patient is operated on, then the higher the success rate. May speed liver transplant.

Further reading

Adear H, Barki Y. Multiseptate gallbladder in a child: incidental diagnosis on sonography. *Pediatr Radiol* 1990; **20**: 192.

Al-Salem AH, Qaisruddin S. The significance of biliary sludge in children with sickle cell disease. *Pediatr Surg Int* 1998; **13(1)**: 14–16.

Applegate KE, Ghei M, Perez-Atayde AR. Prenatal detection of a solitary liver adenoma. *Pediatr Radiol* 1999; **29(2)**: 92–94.

Atkinson GO, Kodroff M, Sones PJ, Gay BB. Focal nodular hyperplasia of the liver in children: a report of three new cases. *Radiology* 1980; **137**: 171–174.

Barzilai M, Lerner A. Gallbladder polyps in children: a rare condition. *Pediatr Radiol* 1997; **27(1)**: 54–56.

Bates SM, Keller MS, Ramos IM, Carter D, Taylor KJ. Hepatoblastoma: detection of tumor vascularity with duplex Doppler US. *Radiology* 1990; **176(2)**: 505–507.

Blickman JG, Herrin JT, Cleveland RH, Jaramillo D. Coexisting nephrolithiasis and cholelithiasis in premature infants. *Pediatr Radiol* 1991; **21**: 363–364.

Callahan J, Haller JO, Cacciarelli AA, Slovis TL, Friedman P. Cholelithiasis in infants: association with total parenteral nutrition and furosemide. *Radiology* 1982; **143**: 437–439.

Chateil J, Brun M, Perel Y, Pillet P, Micheau M, Diard F. Abdominal ultrasound findings in children with hemophagocytic lymphohistiocytosis. *Eur Radiol* 1999; **9(3)**: 474–477.

Davenport M, Stringer MD, Howard ER. Biliary amylase and congenital choledochal dilatation. *J Pediatr Surg* 1995; **30(3)**: 474–477.

Donovan AT, Wolverson MK, deMello D, Craddock T, Silberstein M. Multicystic hepatic mesenchymal hamartoma of childhood. *Pediatr Radiol* 1981; **11**: 163–165.

Engel JM, Deitch EA, Sikkema W. Gallbladder wall thickness: sonographic accuracy and relation to disease. *AJR* 1980; **134**: 907–909.

Federici S, Galli G, Sciutti R, Cuoghi D. Cystic mesenchymal hamartoma of the liver. *Pediatr Radiol* 1992; **22(4)**: 307–308.

Gerhold JP, Klingensmith WC, Kuni CC. Diagnosis of biliary atresia with radionuclide hepatobiliary imaging. *Radiology* 1983; **146**: 499–504.

Greenholz SK, Krishnadasan B, Marr C, Cannon R. Biliary obstruction in infants with cystic fibrosis requiring Kasai portoenterostomy. *J Pediatr Surg* 1997; **32(2)**: 175–179.

Haller JO. Sonography of the biliary tract in infants and children. *AJR* 1991; **157**: 1051–1058.

Han BK, Babcock DS, Gelfand MH. Choledochal cyst with bile duct dilatation: sonography and 99m-Tc IDA cholescintigraphy. *AJR* 1981; **136**: 1075–1079.

Helmberger TK, Ros PR, Mergo PJ, Tomczak R, Reiser MF. Pediatric liver neoplasms: a radiologic-pathologic correlation. *Eur Radiol* 1999; **9(7)**: 1339–1347.

Hernanz-Schulman M, Ambrosino MM, Freeman PC et al. Common bile duct in children: sonographic dimensions. *Radiology* 1995; **195**: 193–195.

Ikeda S, Sera Y, Ohshiro H, Uchino S, Akizuki M, Kondo Y. Gallbladder contraction in biliary atresia: a pitfall of ultrasound diagnosis. *Pediatr Radiol* 1998; **28(6)**: 451–453.

Kurtz AB, Rubin CS, Cooper HS, Nisenbaum HL, Cole-Beuglet C, Medoff J, Goldberg BB. Ultrasound findings in hepatitis. *Radiology* 1980; **136**: 717–723.

Lam AH, Shulman L. Ultrasonography in the management of liver trauma in children. *J Ultrasound Med* 1984; **3**: 199–203.

Marchal GJ, Desmet VJ, Proesmans WC, Moerman PL, Roost WW, Van Holsbeeck MT, Baert AL. Caroli disease: high-frequency US and pathologic findings. *Radiology* 1986; **158**: 507–511.

McGahan JP, Phillips HE, Cox KL. Sonography of the normal pediatric gallbladder and biliary tract. *Radiology* 1982; **144(4)**: 873–875.

Meilstrup JW, Hopper KD, Thieme GA. Imaging of gallbladder variants. *Am J Radiol* 1991; **157**: 1205–1208.

Miller WJ, Sechtin AG, Campbell WL et al. Imaging findings in Caroli's disease. *Am J Radiol* 1995; **165**: 333–337.

Mitchell SE, Gross BH, Spitz HB. The hypoechoic caudate lobe: an ultrasonic pseudolesion. *Radiology* 1982; **144**: 569–572.

Mittelstaedt CA, Volberg FM, Fischer GJ, McCartney WH. Caroli's disease: sonographic findings. *AJR* 1980; **134**: 585–587.

Newlin N, Silver TM, Stuck KJ, Sandler MA. Ultrasonic features of pyogenic liver abscesses. *Radiology* 1981; **139**: 155–159.

Parulekar SG. Ligaments and fissures of the liver: sonographic anatomy. *Radiology* 1979; **130**: 409–411.

Patriquin HB, DePietro M, Barber FE, Teele RL. Sonography of thickened gallbladder wall: causes in children. *AJR* 1983; **141**: 57–60.

Patriquin H, Lafortune M, Burns PN, Dauzat M. Duplex Doppler examination in portal hypertension: technique and anatomy. *AJR* 1987; **149**: 71–76.

Ralls PW, Quinn MF, Boswell WD, Colletti PM, Radin DR, Halls J. Patterns of resolution in successfully treated hepatic amebic abscess: sonographic evaluation. *Radiology* 1983; **149**: 541–543

Rollins NK, Timmons C, Superina RA, Andrews WS. Hepatic artery thrombosis in children with liver transplants: false-positive findings at Doppler sonography and arteriography in four patients. *AJR* 1993; **160**: 291–294.

Ros PR, Goodman ZD, Ishak KG, Dachman AH, Olmsted WW, Hartman DS, Lichtenstein JE. Mesenchymal hamartoma of the liver: radiologic-pathologic correlation. *Radiology* 1986; **158**: 619–624.

Rosenbaum DM, Mindell HJ. Ultrasonographic findings in mesenchymal hamartoma of the liver. *Radiology* 1981; **138**: 425–427.

Roslyn JJ, Berquist WE, Pitt HA, Mann LL, Kangarloo H, DenBesten L, Ament ME. Increased risk of gallstones in children receiving total parenteral nutrition. *Pediatrics* 1983; **71**: 784–789.

Scatarige JC, Scott WW, Donovan PJ, Siegelman SS, Sander RC. Fatty infiltration of the liver: ultrasonographic and computed tomographic correlation. *J Ultrasound Med* 1984; **3**: 9–14.

Senaati S, Gumruk FU, Delbakhsh P, Balkanci F, Altay C. Gallbladder pathology in pediatric beta-thalassemic patients. A prospective ultrasonographic study. *Pediatr Radiol* 1994; **23(5)**: 357–359.

Siegel MJ, Melson GL. Sonographic demonstration of hepatic Burkitt's lymphoma. *Pediatr Radiol* 1981; **11**: 166–167.

Soucy P, Rasuli P, Chou S, Carpenter B. Definitive treatment of focal nodular hyperplasia of the liver by ethanol embolization. *J Pediatr Surg* 1989; **24(10)**: 1095–1097.

Subramanyam BR, Balthazar EJ, Madamba MR, Raghavendra BN, Horii SC, Lefleur RS. Sonography of portosystemic venous collaterals in portal hypertension. *Radiology* 1983; **146**: 161–166.

Tessler FN, Gehring BJ, Gomes AS, *et al*. Diagnosis of portal vein thrombosis: value of color Doppler imaging. *AJR* 1991; **157**: 293–296.

Toma P, Lucigrai G, Pelizza A. Sonographic patterns of Caroli's disease: report of 5 new cases. *J Clin Ultrasound* 1991; **19**: 155–161.

Torrisi JM, Haller JO, Velcek FT. Choledochal cyst and biliary atresia in the neonate: imaging findings in five cases. *AJR* 1990; **155**: 1273–1276.

Welch TJ, Sheedy PF II, Johnson CM, *et al*. Focal nodular hyperplasia and hepatic adenoma: comparison of angiography, CT, US, and scintigraphy. *Radiology* 1985; **156**: 593–595.

Weltin G, Taylor KJW, Carter AR, Taylor CR. Duplex Doppler: identification of cavernous transformation of the portal vein. *AJR* 1985; **144**: 999–1001.

Westra SJ, Zaninovic AC, Hall TR, Busuttil RW, Kangarloo H, Boechat MI. Imaging in pediatric liver transplantation. *Radiographics* 1994; **13(5)**: 1081–1099.

Wholey MH, Wojno KJ. Pediatric hepatic mesenchymal hamartoma demonstrated on plain film, ultrasound and MRI, and correlated with pathology. *Pediatr Radiol* 1994; **24(2)**: 143–144.

Wozney P, Zajko AB, Bron KM, Point S, Starzl TE. Vascular complications after liver transplantation: a 5-year experience. *AJR* 1986; **147**: 657–663.

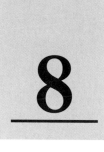

8

THE
PANCREAS

The pancreas lies in the retroperitoneum, posterior to the left lobe of liver and stomach. The head of pancreas lies in the curve of the duodenum, the body and tail obliquely to the left over the splenic vein, the tail extending to the splenic hilum. Vascular landmarks which help to locate the pancreas include the aorta, superior mesenteric artery (SMA), superior mesenteric vein (SMV) and splenic vein. Non-vascular landmarks are the pancreatic duct and common duct (Fig. 8.1).

TRANSDUCER

Highest frequency curvilinear transducer possible depending on patient build.

PREPARATION

In general no preparation, but if the patient is fasted this should help reduce bowel gas.

TECHNIQUE

Patient lies supine. Transducer is placed in the epigastric region in the midline inferior to the xiphisternum and is moved gently caudally to identify the landmarks if not found easily. Oblique sections may be required to demonstrate the length of the gland, although the tail may be obscured by overlying bowel gas (see technique for overcoming bowel gas in this section). The transducer is then rotated through 90 degrees and the gland assessed in sequential parasagittal sections.

Table 8.1 Normal dimensions of the pancreas as a function of age

Patient age	No. of patients	Maximum anteroposterior dimensions of pancreas (cm ± 1 standard deviation)		
		Head	Body	Tail
<1 mo	15	1.0 ± 0.4	0.6 ± 0.2	1.0 ± 0.4
1 mo–1 yr	23	1.5 ± 0.5	0.8 ± 0.3	1.2 ± 0.4
1–5 yr	49	1.7 ± 0.3	1.0 ± 0.2	1.8 ± 0.4
5–10 yr	69	1.6 ± 0.4	1.0 ± 0.3	1.8 ± 0.4
10–19 yr	117	2.0 ± 0.5	1.1 ± 0.3	2.0 ± 0.4

As published in Siegel MJ, Martin KW, Worthington JL. Normal and abnormal pancreas in children: US studies. *Radiology* 1987; **165**: 15–18.

Normal ultrasound appearances

- Comma-shaped with a smooth outline (Fig. 8.2).

- Homogeneous in echotexture.

- Similar echogenicity or slightly less echogenic than adjacent liver.

- Pancreatic size varies with age (Table 8.1).

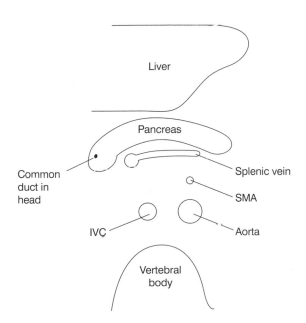

Figure 8.1 — Transverse section through the upper abdomen demonstrating the anatomical landmarks used to identify the pancreas.

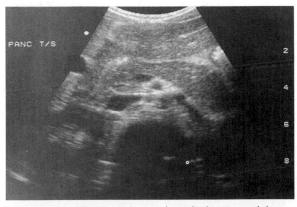

Figure 8.2 — Transverse section through the upper abdomen showing the normal body and tail of pancreas surrounding the superior mesenteric artery and vein.

- The normal pancreatic duct can be seen with a high frequency transducer and measures 1–2mm, and appears as either:
  - an echogenic line running through the centre of the body of pancreas, or
  - two parallel lines with an echofree space between (Fig. 8.3).

Techniques for overcoming bowel gas

Application of gentle transducer pressure to displace bowel gas.

Change of patient position, e.g.

Prone – left kidney can be used as an acoustic window to assess the tail.

Erect – bowel loops displaced inferiorly under the influence of gravity.

Right decubitus position – to aid visualisation of the head.

Change in respiratory phase, e.g. deep inspiration or ask children to push their tummy out.

Fluid loading. Fluid is administered via a straw, in the right decubitus position. The stomach can then be used as an acoustic window.

Pancreatic anomalies

Pancreas divisum

This is the most common pancreatic anomaly. It results from failure of fusion of the ventral and dorsal portions which are drained by separate ducts that do not communicate. Not usually demonstrable ultrasonically.

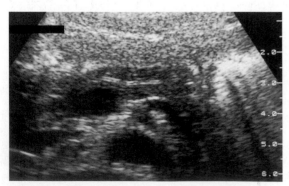

Figure 8.3 — Normal pancreatic duct. Note echogenic parallel lines in the body of the pancreas.

Annular pancreas

Results from the development of bifid ventral buds which encircle the duodenum as they move to fuse with the dorsal bud.

ASSOCIATED ANOMALIES

Duodenal stenosis

Duodenal atresia.

Ultrasound demonstrates a solid band of pancreatic tissue around the duodenum but not always identifiable.

Short pancreas

Associated with polysplenia.

A rounded pancreas is seen adjacent to the duodenum.

Pancreatitis

Acute

Oedematous swelling of the pancreas associated with abdominal pain and sometimes transient jaundice.

Uncommon in children.

CAUSES

Post trauma – typically handlebar injury or knee in epigastrium. Always consider NAI in the young child.

Virus infection.

Drug toxicity.

Occasionally cholelithiasis.

ULTRASOUND APPEARANCES – VARIABLE

- May appear normal in early stages.
- Homogeneous echotexture.
- Enlarged gland – diffuse or focal.
- Hypoechoic in comparison to the liver.
- Dilated pancreatic duct is sometimes seen (Fig. 8.4).
- Fluid collections: either peripancreatic, pancreatic pseudocyst or fluid in the peritoneal cavity.
- Associated dilatation of the biliary tree due to compression of the CBD by the swollen head.

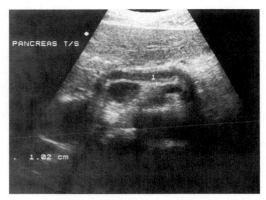

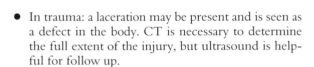

Figure 8.4 — Dilated duct within the body of the pancreas, post traumatic pancreatitis.

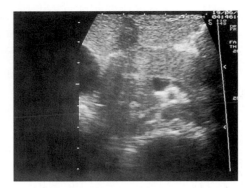

Figure 8.5 — Chronic pancreatitis. Note enlarged amorphous pancreas.

- In trauma: a laceration may be present and is seen as a defect in the body. CT is necessary to determine the full extent of the injury, but ultrasound is helpful for follow up.

Chronic

Repeated attacks of pancreatitis result in chronic changes: fibrosis, calcification and calculi.

CLINICAL PRESENTATION

Hereditary pancreatitis, an autosomal dominant disorder, results in repeated attacks of acute pancreatitis which often begin in childhood.

Anomalies: annular pancreas, pancreatic divisum.

Cystic fibrosis.

Idiopathic pancreatitis.

Malnutrition.

ULTRASOUND APPEARANCES
Early stages
- Enlargement (Fig. 8.5).
- Hypoechoic.
- Duct dilatation.

As condition progresses
- Heterogeneous echotexture.
- Focal/diffuse enlargement with areas of increased echogenicity.

- Pseudocysts.
- Calcification and calculi may occur.

Late stages
- Atrophic, fibrosed.
- Small, echogenic gland with heterogeneous echotexture.
- Dilated pancreatic duct which can appear beaded.
- Dilatation of the extrahepatic biliary tree due to compression of the common bile duct by the fibrotic gland.

Cystic fibrosis (CF)

An hereditary disease due to an autosomal recessive gene, causing glandular secretions to be excessively viscous. Affects approximately 1 in 2000 children in the UK.

CLINICAL PRESENTATION

Usually examined as part of the routine annual review of patients with CF. Clinical presentation of pancreatitis in CF patients is rare.

ULTRASOUND APPEARANCES
- Increased echogenicity compared to adjacent liver (assuming normal liver), but the liver is often heterogeneous due to CF liver disease (Fig. 8.6).

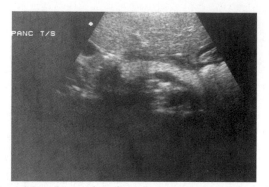

Figure 8.6 — Hyperechoic featureless pancreas in a patient with cystic fibrosis.

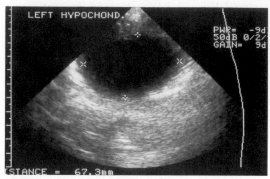

Figure 8.8 — Large well-defined cystic mass in the left hypochondrium arising in the tail of the pancreas.

- Small cysts (Fig. 8.7).
- Calcification.
- Atrophy.

Pancreatic cysts

Uncommon.

Pseudocysts

Seen in acute and chronic pancreatitis.

ULTRASOUND APPEARANCES (Fig. 8.8)
- Thin-walled.
- Well defined.
- Anechoic.
- May contain internal echoes with a fluid/debris level.

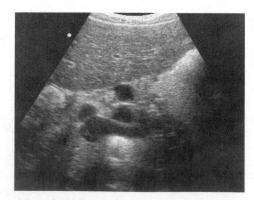

Figure 8.7 — Multiple cysts in the pancreas.

- Unilocular or multilocular.
- May be quite large. Can extend into the mediastinum.
- Acoustic enhancement.

Congenital cysts

Usually asymptomatic.

Seen in association with polycystic disease and Von Hippel-Lindau disease. Can only be differentiated from a pseudocyst on clinical grounds.

ULTRASOUND APPEARANCES
Thin-walled, well-defined, anechoic lesions which demonstrate cystic enhancement.

Pancreatic tumours

Rare in childhood.

Classified into exocrine and endocrine tumours.

Non-functioning tumours

- Adenocarcinoma – aggressive tumour arising in the pancreatic head, which has often spread at the time of diagnosis.
- Pancreatoblastoma – occurs in infancy and has a good prognosis. Usually well-defined. Arises in the pancreatic head.
- Lymphangioma.
- Hamartoma.
- Sarcoma (Fig. 8.9).

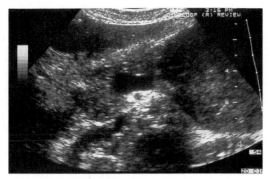

Figure 8.9 — Sarcoma of the pancreas. Note enlarged irregular mixed echo mass.

- Lymphoma (Fig. 8.10).
- Haemangioendothelioma.

Functioning tumours/Islet cell tumours

Insulinoma.

Gastrinoma.

VIP oma (Vasoactive Intestinal Polypeptide).

The diagnosis is confirmed by hormone assay.

Usually small < 2 cm in diameter.

Those tumours that are hormonally inactive present only when symptoms occur due to their size.

CLINICAL PRESENTATION

Abdominal pain.

Palpable mass.

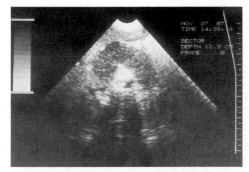

Figure 8.10 — Pancreatic lymphoma. The gland is enlarged and featureless.

ULTRASOUND APPEARANCES

- Focal or diffuse mass.
- Majority hypoechoic in comparison to surrounding pancreatic tissue, but can be isoechoic, hyperechoic.
- Calcification.
- Cysts.
- Usually well-defined.
- May or may not see dilatation of the biliary tree, and/or pancreatic duct.
- Assessment should include a search for evidence of spread: liver, porta hepatis, and adjacent retroperitoneum.

Nesidioblastomatosis

A diffuse insulin secreting tumour of the pancreas in the neonatal period leading to profound hypoglycaemia. Ultrasonic appearances are normal.

Further reading

Atkinson GO Jr, Wyly JB, Gay BB Jr, Ball TI, Winn JK. Idiopathic fibrosing pancreatitis: a cause of obstructive jaundice in childhood. *Pediatr Radiol* 1988; **18**: 28–31.

Daneman A, Gaskin K, Martin DJ, Cutz E. Pancreatic changes in cystic fibrosis: CT and sonographic appearances. *AJR* 1983; **141**: 653–655.

Gorenstein A, O'Halpin D, Wesson DE, Daneman A, Filler RM. Blunt injury to the pancreas in children: selective management based on ultrasound. *J Pediatr Surg* 1987; **22**: 1110–1116.

Hadar H, Gadoth N, Herskovitz P, Heifetz M. Short pancreas in polysplenia syndrome. *Acta Radiol* 1991; **32**: 299–301.

Herman TE, Siegel MJ. Polysplenia syndrome with congenital short pancreas. *AJR* 1991; **156**: 799–800.

Jeffrey RB Jr. Sonography in acute pancreatitis. *Radiol Clin North Am* 1989; **27**: 5–17.

McHugo JM, McKeown C, Brown MT, Weller P, Shah KJ. Ultrasound findings in children with cystic fibrosis. *Br J Radiol* 1987; **60**: 137–141.

Ros PR, Hamrick-Turner JE, Chiechi MV, Ros LH, Gallego P, Burton SS. Cystic masses of the pancreas. *Radiographics* 1992; **12**: 673–686.

Siegel MJ, Martin KW, Worthington JL. Normal and abnormal pancreas in children: US studies. *Radiology* 1987; **165**: 15–18.

Willi UV, Reddish JM, Teele RL. Cystic fibrosis: its characteristic appearance on abdominal sonography. *AJR* 1980; **134**: 1005–1010.

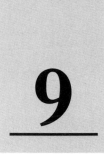

9

THE
SPLEEN

Lies superiorly to the left kidney beneath the left hemi-diaphragm, laterally to the adrenal and tail of pancreas and posterior to the left hemi-diaphragm. The splenic artery and vein enter the medical aspect of the spleen at the splenic hilum.

PREPARATION

None required.

TRANSDUCER

Highest frequency curvilinear transducer compatible with the patient's build.

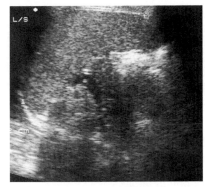

Figure 9.1 — Normal appearance of the spleen in the long axis.

TECHNIQUE

Patient lies in the right decubitus position. The spleen rotates anteriorly and inferiorly and therefore more of the spleen is demonstrated below the costal margin. The transducer is placed in the 10th/11th intercostal space providing a coronal section. Anteroposterior angulation allows visualisation of the entire spleen in coronal section. The transducer is then rotated through 90 degrees, and angled superiorly and inferiorly to image the spleen in sequential transverse sections.

PROBLEMS

Limited access due to overlying rib cage and narrow intercostal spaces; overcome by placing a pillow/foam pad under the patient's waist and placing the left arm up close to the patient's head.

Deep inspiration may result in descent of the lung over the spleen posteriorly and laterally therefore reducing its visualisation, for optimum view encourage quiet respiration.

Normal ultrasound appearances

(Fig. 9.1)

- Crescent-shaped.

- Homogeneous echotexture.

- More echogenic than adjacent kidney.

- Similar or slightly more echogenic than the liver at the same depth.

- Size varies with age (Table 9.1).

Table 9.1 Age and splenic length in 230 infants and children

Age (Number)	Length of Spleen (cm)			
	10th %ile	Median	90th %ile	Suggested upper limit
0–3 months (n = 28)	3.3	4.5	5.8	6.0
3–6 months (n = 13)	4.9	5.3	6.4	6.5
6–12 months (n = 17)	5.2	6.2	6.8	7.0
1–2 years (n = 12)	5.4	6.9	7.5	8.0
2–4 years (n = 24)	6.4	7.4	8.6	9.0
4–6 years (n = 39)	6.9	7.8	8.8	9.5
6–8 years (n = 21)	7.0	8.2	9.6	10.0
8–10 years (n = 16)	7.9	9.2	10.5	11.0
10–12 years (n = 17)	8.6	9.9	10.9	11.5
12–15 years (n = 26)	8.7	10.1	11.4	12.0
15–20 years (n = 17)				
Female	9.0	10.0	11.7	12.0
Male	10.1	11.2	12.6	13.0

From Rosenberg et al 1991.

Splenic anomalies

Asplenia

Absence of splenic tissue.

More common in males.

Associated with severe cardiac anomalies.

Polysplenia

Multiple aberrant nodules of splenic tissue.

More common in females.

ASSOCIATED ANOMALIES

Mild cardiac anomalies

Dextrocardia

Malrotation.

Accessory spleen (Fig. 9.2)

Seen in approximately 5% of children.

Oval or round structure, identical in echotexture to the spleen, found at the hilum or inferior pole of the spleen approximately 1 cm in diameter.

Usually an incidental finding and of no consequence.

Wandering spleen

An ectopically located spleen, due to a deficiency in ligament attachments or an abnormally long pedicle.

CLINICAL PRESENTATION

Abdominal mass.

Acute/chronic torsion.

Situs invertus

The spleen is located on the right side of the abdomen.

Splenomegaly (Fig. 9.3)

Enlargement of the spleen.

CLINICAL PRESENTATION

Palpable mass.

ASSOCIATED WITH

Malignant disease

Inflammatory disease

Infection

Lymphadenopathy

Lymphoma

Portal hypertension

Mass lesions within the spleen, e.g. abscess, metastases, cysts.

ULTRASOUND APPEARANCES

- Enlarged.
- Loss of normal concavity.
- Normal echotexture.
- Focal involvement, eg. metastases, cysts, abscess.

Splenic cysts

Uncommon in children.

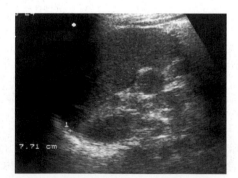

Figure 9.2 — An area of accessory splenic tissue lying under the normal spleen.

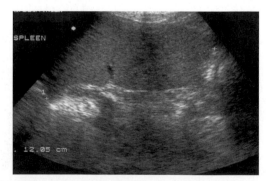

Figure 9.3 — An enlarged spleen measuring 12 cm in an 8-year-old child with leukaemia.

Classified as:

I. True cysts

Usually congenital epidermoid, lined with epithelium and having fibrous walls (Figs. 9.4, 9.5).

II. False cysts:

Usually a result of trauma, infection, ischaemia.

Parasitic (due to hydatid disease) or non-parasitic in origin.

CLINICAL PRESENTATION

Palpable LUQ mass.

Pain due to mass effect on other organs.

Acute pain due to haemorrhage or infection within the cyst.

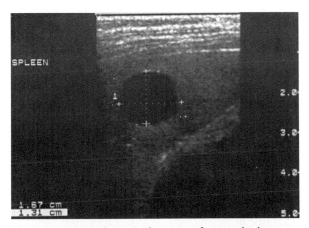

Figure 9.4 — A simple cyst in the centre of a normal spleen.

ULTRASOUND APPEARANCES

- Anechoic with post-cystic enhancement.

- Well-defined, usually spherical.

- Internal echoes are present with haemorrhage and infection (Fig. 9.6).

- Parasitic cysts may contain daughter cysts and septations.

- Sometimes have calcification.

Abscesses

Uncommon.

Usually solitary.

Usually due to haematogenous spread of infection, trauma or infarction.

CLINICAL PRESENTATION

Fever.

LUQ tenderness.

Splenomegaly.

ULTRASOUND APPEARANCES

- Hypoechoic lesion with some posterior enhancement.

- Irregular outline, often thick-walled.

- May contain internal echoes, fluid–debris level.

- If it contains a gas-forming organism echogenic foci with ill-defined acoustic shadowing may be seen.

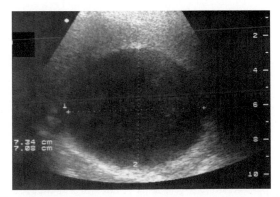

Figure 9.5 — Large splenic cyst compressing normal tissue so the normal spleen is not visible.

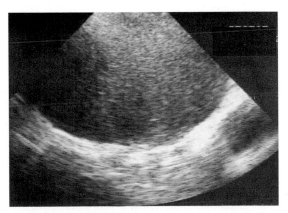

Figure 9.6 — Large splenic cyst with echogenic fluid due to haemorrhage.

Splenic infarction

A result of occlusion of the splenic artery or one of its branches.

May occur as a complication of:

– leukaemia

– sickle cell anaemia

– bacterial endocarditis

– splenomegaly.

CLINICAL PRESENTATION

Acutely painful left upper quadrant.

ULTRASOUND APPEARANCES

● Variable.

● Initially may appear normal.

● During the acute phase: wedge-shaped hypoechoic area which becomes more hyperechoic and may atrophy leaving an echogenic scar.

● Repeated infarcts result in a small spleen with multiple echogenic areas representing old infarcts or a diffusely echogenic spleen.

Trauma

Usually a result of blunt abdominal trauma.

Examination can be difficult due to pain and bowel gas.

Classified as:

– haematomas

– lacerations

– fractures

– subcapsular collections.

CLINICAL PRESENTATION

Blunt abdominal injury.

LUQ tenderness.

ULTRASOUND APPEARANCES (Fig. 9.7)

● Haematomas

– variable

– initially hypoechoic/isoechoic to normal splenic tissue; as lysis occurs hypoechoic. Complete

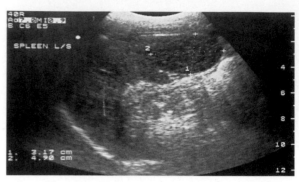

Figure 9.7— Following trauma to the abdomen an hypoechoic area is demonstrated at the lower pole of the spleen, the remainder is normal in echotexture.

resolution usually occurs within 1 year; a residual scar may be seen as a linear echogenic focus.

● Lacerations

– usually involve lateral margins

– irregular linear lesions.

● Fractures involve splenic hilum.

● Subcapsular collections are crescent-shaped and may cause alteration in splenic outline. Free fluid is seen and there is capsular disruption.

Lymphoma

Enlarged spleen.

Loss of normal echotexture with heterogeneous appearance.

Occasionally discrete deposits (Fig. 9.8).

Usually associated with nodal disease.

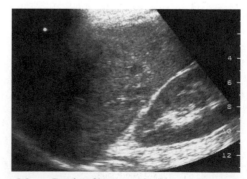

Figure 9.8 — Focal infiltration of spleen in Non-Hodgkin's lymphoma. Note irregular echotexture with small hypoechoic deposits.

Further reading

Chew FS, Smith PL, Barboriak D. Candidal splenic abscesses. *AJR* 1991; **156**: 474

Daneman A, Martin DJ. Congenital epithelial splenic cysts in children. Emphasis on sonographic appearances and some unusual features. *Pediatr Radiol* 1982; **12**: 119–125.

Dittrich M, Milde S, Dinkel E, Baumann W, Weitzel D. Sonographic biometry of liver and spleen size in childhood. *Pediatr Radiol* 1983; **13**: 206–211.

George C, Schwerk WB. Splenic infarction: sonographic patterns, diagnosis, follow–up, and complications. *Radiology* 1990; **174**: 803–807.

George C, Schwerk WB, Goerg K, Havemann K. Sonographic patterns of the affected spleen in malignant lymphoma. *J Clin Ultrasound* 1990; **18**: 569–574.

Goske Rudick M, Wood BP, Lerner RM. Splenic abscess diagnosed by ultrasound in the pediatric patient. Report of three cases. *Pediatr Radiol* 1983; **13**: 269–271.

Herman TE, Siegel MJ. CT of acute splenic torsion in children with wandering spleen. *AJR* 1991; **156**: 151–153.

Rosenberg HK, Markowitz RI, Kolberg H, Park C, Hubbard A, Bellah RD. Normal splenic size in infants and children: sonographic measurements. *AJR* 1991; **157**: 119–121.

10

THE
ADRENALS

Anteromedial to the upper poles of both kidneys. Each gland has a central body directed anteromedially and two limbs directed posterolaterally. Typically 'V' or 'Y'-shaped.

PREPARATION

None necessary, but fasting for 6–8 hours may reduce food residue and overlying bowel gas.

TRANSDUCER

High frequency curvilinear transducer. Highest frequency compatible with patient build.

TECHNIQUE

The right adrenal is imaged with the patient supine, using the liver as an acoustic window. Slight medial angulation may be required. The left adrenal is imaged with the patient in the right decubitus position. The left kidney is identified in the long axis and then slight medial angulation will demonstrate the adrenal using the spleen and left kidney as an acoustic window.

Normal ultrasound appearances

- Typically 'V' or 'Y'-shaped. (Figs. 10.1, 10.2).

- Appearances vary with age.

- In neonates: hyperechoic centre (medulla) and hypoechoic rim (cortex).

- Gradually increase in echogenicity and by 1 year are similar to the adult gland.

- Hyperechoic with loss of differentiation between the medulla and cortex.

NB. The crescent or triangular hyperechoic structure found superior to the kidney is perirenal fat not the adrenal.

Anomalies of the adrenal gland

Absence

Rare.

Associated with renal agenesis.

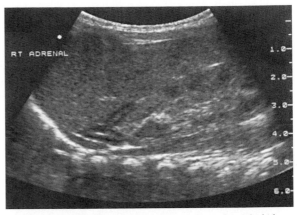

Figure 10.1 — Normal right adrenal seen above the right kidney. Note Y-shaped configuration.

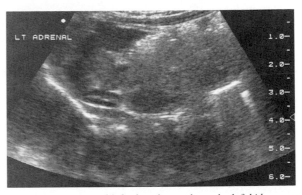

Figure 10.2 — Normal left adrenal seen above the left kidney.

Hypoplasia

Occurs in anencephalic infants.

ASSOCIATED ANOMALIES

Severe hydrocephalus

Neonatal adrenoleukodystrophy

Zellweger's syndrome.

Fusion

2 types:

(1) Fusion of the two wings producing a circular gland

(2) Fusion of right and left adrenal glands producing a horseshoe

ASSOCIATED ANOMALIES

Horseshoe kidney

Asplenia.

Adrenal haemorrhage

Usually occurs in neonates.

Most common cause of adrenal mass in a neonate.

Occurs unilaterally or bilaterally.

Associated with birth trauma and perinatal asphyxia.

Trauma and meningitis can cause adrenal haemorrhage in older children.

CLINICAL PRESENTATION

Abdominal mass.

Anaemia.

Jaundice.

Vomiting.

Hypertension.

Intestinal obstruction.

Impaired renal function.

Renal vein thrombosis.

ULTRASOUND APPEARANCES (Fig. 10.3)

• Depends on the extent and age of the haemorrhage.

• Large lesions are usually spherical, small ones triangular or crescent-shaped.

• Initially appears as a highly echogenic mass above the kidney.

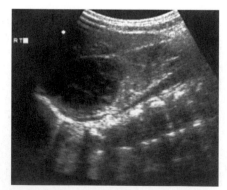

Figure 10.3 — Neonatal adrenal haemorrhage seen as a large cystic mass above the right kidney.

• After 1–2 weeks appears as a complex mass (liquefaction occurs) decreasing in size and eventually completely cystic.

• After resolution a residual focus of calcification is sometimes seen (Fig. 10.4).

PITFALLS

Can be difficult to differentiate from a neuroblastoma initially, but after 1–2 weeks a neuroblastoma remains echogenic and continues to increase in size.

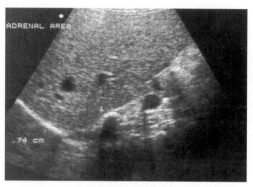

Figure 10.4 — Calcification within the right adrenal gland secondary to haemorrhage in the neonatal period. Note acoustic shadow.

Adrenal abscess

Rare.

Occurs unilaterally or bilaterally.

Often develops as a complication of adrenal haemorrhage.

CLINICAL PRESENTATION

Suprarenal mass.

ULTRASOUND APPEARANCES

Hypoechoic with internal echoes/debris.

May demonstrate fluid/debris levels.

Occasionally appears solid.

PITFALLS

Again can be difficult to distinguish from adrenal haemorrhage or neuroblastoma. An increase in size together with a fever is most likely to represent an abscess.

TREATMENT

Early diagnosis and treatment is necessary to prevent complications. Often requires surgery.

Adrenal cysts

True simple cysts are rare (Fig. 10.5).

Usually asymptomatic.

Associated with Beckwith Weidemann syndrome.

Pseudocysts are seen as a result of resolving haemorrhage. The history of such a haemorrhage distinguishes a pseudocyst from a simple cyst.

ULTRASOUND APPEARANCES

- Well-defined, usually spherical in shape.
- Anechoic.
- Demonstrate post cystic enhancement.
- Occasionally may appear complex, and contain septae or debris.

Tumours

Neuroblastoma

Most common adrenal tumour.

Usually occurs in children < 4 years.

Majority of tumours arise in the adrenal but can originate anywhere along the sympathetic chain. Tumours in the chest have a better prognosis.

CLINICAL PRESENTATION

Palpable abdominal mass.

Fever.

Loss of weight.

Irritability.

Hypertension.

Anaemia.

Bone pain.

The tumours tend to be aggressive in nature and metastasise early and therefore a child may present with symptoms due to metastases.

ULTRASOUND APPEARANCES

- Suprarenal mass displacing the kidney.
- Poorly defined margins.
- Variable echotexture
  - usually mainly solid. Cystic varieties are rare.
  - heterogeneous – hyper/hypoechoic areas (Fig. 10.6).
  - calcification – echogenic foci in the tumour. Acoustic shadowing unusual as foci are small.
  - anechoic areas – necrosis.
  - haemorrhage.
- Often encases major vessels, displaces and occludes the IVC. Colour Doppler is helpful.
- Liver metastases.
- Nodal disease is usually present but is difficult to distinguish from the primary lesion.

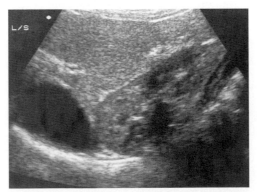

Figure 10.5 — A cystic lesion is demonstrated superior to the upper pole of the left kidney – no normal adrenal tissue is seen. No history of neonatal haemorrhage. Diagnosis – simple adrenal cyst.

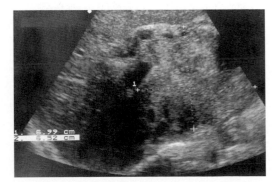

Figure 10.6 — A large ill-defined heterogeneous mass is demonstrated.

LIMITATIONS

The stage of the disease at diagnosis affects the prognosis. MRI and CT are required to determine the full extent of the disease.

Stage IV S neuroblastoma is a rare form, presenting in very young infants.

- Enlarged liver due to metastases.
- Primary often difficult to find or is a small tumour in the adrenals.
- Prognosis is better than classic Stage IV.

Ganglion neuroma (Benign)/ganglion neuroblastoma

(Variable spectrum from almost benign to aggressive)

Two more benign tumours which arise in the adrenals or sympathetic chain.

Similar ultrasonic appearances to neuroblastoma.

Ganglion neuroma is well defined.

Adrenal carcinoma

Arises in the adrenal cortex.

CLINICAL PRESENTATION

Usually with endocrine effects, e.g. Cushing's syndrome, or precocious puberty.

ULTRASOUND APPEARANCES

- Solid mass in suprarenal region (Fig. 10.7).
- Calcification variable but not prominent.

- Usually well circumscribed.
- Nodes, if present, indicate malignancy.

Metastasises to liver and lungs and adjacent nodes.

Phaeochromocytoma

Rare.

Usually benign but < 10% are malignant.

Can be hereditary.

ASSOCIATED ANOMALIES

Neurofibromatosis

Tuberous sclerosis

Von Hippel-Lindau.

CLINICAL PRESENTATION

Hypertension.

Raised urinary catecholamines.

Rarely a palpable mass.

ULTRASOUND APPEARANCES

- Solid – usually homogeneous in echotexture (Fig. 10.8).
- Well-defined, often oval.
- Usually more echogenic than renal parenchyma.
- Calcification occasionally seen.

LIMITATIONS

Biochemical tests are required as it is difficult to distinguish from other tumours with ultrasound.

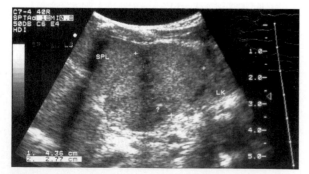

Figure 10.7 — Adrenal carcinoma. A well defined solid mass is demonstrated between the left kidney and spleen.

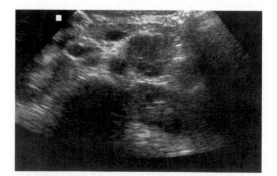

Figure 10.8 — Transverse section left kidney area with a phaeochromocytoma near the tail of the pancreas.

Congenital Adrenal Hyperplasia

Autosomal recessive disorder.

Due to an enzyme deficiency.

CLINICAL PRESENTATION

Virilism in newborn females.

Early masculinisation in boys.

Ambiguous genitalia.

ULTRASOUND APPEARANCES (Fig. 10.9)

- Usually enlarged – adrenals appear more triangular and irregular in outline.

- May be normal, or at upper limit in size.

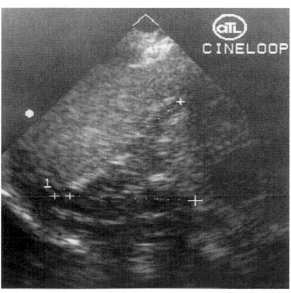

Figure 10.9 — An enlarged adrenal gland.

Further reading

Amundson GM, Trevenen CL, Mueller DL, Rubin SZ, Wesenberg RL. Neuroblastoma: a specific sonographic tissue pattern. *AJR* 1987; **148**: 943–945.

Avni EF, Rypens F, Smet MH, Galetty E. Sonographic demonstration of congenital adrenal hyperplasia in the neonate: the cerebriform pattern. *Pediatr Radiol* 1993; **23**: 88–90.

Berdon WE, Ruzal-Shapiro C, Abramson SJ, Garvin J. The diagnosis of abdominal neuroblastoma: relative roles of ultrasonography, CT, and MRI. *Urol Radiol* 1992; **14**: 252–262.

Black J, Williams DI. Natural history of adrenal haemorrhage in the newborn. *Arch Dis Child* 1973; **48**: 183–190.

Bryan PJ, Caldamone AA, Morrison SC, Yulish BS, Owens R. Ultrasound findings in the adreno-genital syndrome (congenital adrenal hyperplasia). *J Ultrasound Med* 1988; **7**: 675–679.

Carty A, Stanley P. Bilateral adrenal abscesses in a neonate. *Pediatr Radiol* 1973; **1**: 63–64.

Croitoru DP, Sinsky AB, Laberge JM. Cystic neuroblastoma. *J Pediatr Surg* 1992; **27**: 1320–1321.

Daneman A. Adrenal neoplasms in children. *Semin Roentgenol* 1988; **23**: 205–215.

Lee W, Comstock CH, Jurcak-Zaleski S. Prenatal diagnosis of adrenal hemorrhage by ultrasonography. *J Ultrasound Med* 1992; **11**: 369–371.

Levin TL, Morton E. Adrenal hemorrhage complicating ACTH therapy in Crohn's disease. *Pediatr Radiol* 1993; **23**: 457–458.

White SJ, Stuck KJ, Blane CE, Silver TM. Sonography of neuroblastoma. *AJR* 1983; **141**: 465–468.

Wright NB, Smith C, Rickwood AMK, Carty HML. Review imaging children with ambiguous genitalia and intersex states. *Clinical Radiology* 1995; **50**: 823–829.

11

THE RENAL TRACT

CHOICE OF TRANSDUCER

A range of probes are required. The choice depends on the patient size.

GUIDE

Neonates – age 3:   4–7.5 MHz curvilinear.
                     Phased array and linear probes are helpful in infants.
3–10: 4–7.5 MHz curvilinear
10+ : 3–5 MHz curvilinear.

PATIENT PREPARATION

Fluids should be given unless contraindicated by pre-operative restrictions.

TECHNIQUE

If possible, warm the jelly to avoid distressing the child. Start with the bladder, examining it in longitudinal and transverse sections. Assess bladder wall thickness, which should be < 3 mm, and the presence of any ureteric dilatation.

Both kidneys should be examined in sequential longitudinal and transverse sections. The right is usually best imaged in supine and LPO, the left in RPO and right decubitus positions. Where appropriate, pre and post micturition bladder volumes should be measured.

PITFALLS

A distended bladder in a child may cause transient dilatation of the distal ureters which resolve with bladder emptying. If lower ureteric dilatation is seen, the patient must be re-examined post voiding.

A normal variant of configuration of the proximal collecting system is an extrarenal pelvis. This must not be confused with hydronephrosis. In hydronephrosis there is dilatation of both renal pelvis and calyces. There is no dilatation of the calyces with an extrarenal pelvis. A normal extrarenal pelvis will measure no more than 10 mm in transverse diameter.

Renal – normal appearances

In neonates the renal cortex appears as echogenic or more echogenic than the liver/spleen. The renal pyramids appear hypoechoic and are prominent. Care should be taken not to confuse them with cysts. (Fig. 11.1a).

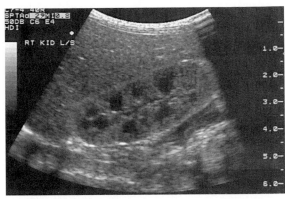

Figure 11.1a — Neonatal kidney. A normal right kidney in a 5-day-old child, the cortex is similar in echogenicity to the liver and the prominent pyramids appear hypoechoic.

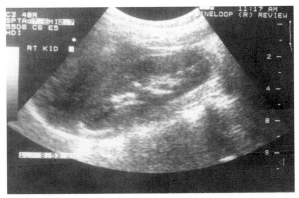

Figure 11.1b — Right kidney. Normal appearance. Note the echogenic renal sinus centrally.

After approximately 3 months of age the kidney is more 'adult' in its appearance with renal cortex slightly less echogenic than the liver/spleen and hypoechoic pyramids surrounding the central sinus echo. (Fig. 11.1b).

Renal length varies with age (Table 11.1)

Normal variants

Fetal lobulation (Fig. 11.2a)
The kidney appears lobulated. This can be differentiated from renal scarring as the indentations occur between renal pyramids. Scarring occurs over renal pyramids, and there is loss of renal cortical depth.

Inter-ranicular septum (Fig. 11.2b)
A linear echogenic defect seen more commonly on the right side.

Table 11.1: Summary of grouped observations – mean renal length

Average Age*	Interval*	Mean Renal Length (cm)	SD	n
0 mo	0–1 wk	4.48	0.31	20
2 mo	1 wk–4 mo	5.28	.66	54
6 mo	4–8 mo	6.15	.67	20
10 mo	8 mo–1 yr	6.23	.63	8
1½	1–2	6.65	.54	28
2½	2–3	7.36	.54	12
3½	3–4	7.36	.64	30
4½	4–5	7.87	.50	26
5½	5–6	8.09	.54	30
6½	6–7	7.83	.72	14
7½	7–8	8.33	.51	18
8½	8–9	8.90	.88	18
9½	9–10	9.20	.90	14
10½	10–11	9.17	.82	28
11½	11–12	9.60	.64	22
12½	12–13	10.42	.87	18
13½	13–14	9.79	.75	14
14½	14–15	10.05	.62	14
15½	15–16	10.93	.76	6
16½	16–17	10.04	.86	10
17½	17–18	10.53	.29	4
18½	18–19	10.81	1.13	8

* Years unless specified otherwise.
Reproduced from Rosenbaum et al AJR: 142, March 1984, 467–469.

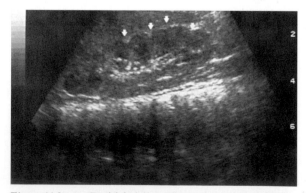

Figure 11.2a — Fetal lobulation. The outline of the kidney is lobulated with the indentations (arrows) between renal pyramids.

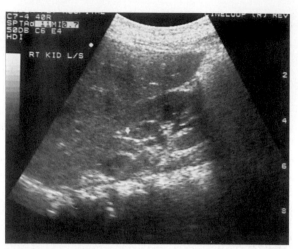

Figure 11.2b — Inter-ranicular septum. A linear echogenic defect (arrow) is shown in the upper pole of the right kidney.

Functional parenchymal defect
A wedge of echogenic tissue, most commonly seen on the supero-anterior surface of the right kidney.

Column of Bertin
An increase in the amount of renal cortex seen between the pyramids. Can be easily distinguished from a mass as it produces no abnormality in the renal outline.

Shape
The left kidney may be squashed by the spleen causing a flattened or distorted outline so that the lateral border bulges – 'dromedary hump'.

Normal Doppler imaging

Renal arteries

Arise from the aorta, and are posteriorly located passing behind the IVC. The typical waveform for a normal renal artery is seen in Fig. 11.3a. A prominent systolic peak followed by a gradual descent to a continuous diastolic flow. The Resistive index of a normal renal artery is < 0.7.

Renal veins

Connect the kidneys to the IVC and lie anterior to the renal arteries. The typical continuous waveform of a normal renal vein is seen in Fig. 11.3b. Respiration may cause minor fluctuations in velocities.

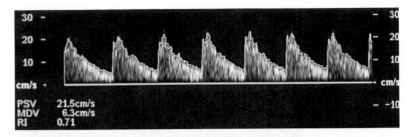

Figure 11.3a — The normal renal artery waveform with a prominent systolic peak followed by gradual descent to a continuous diastolic flow.

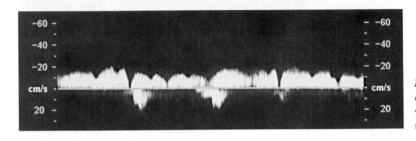

Figure 11.3b — The normal renal vein demonstrating a continuous waveform but with minor fluctuations in velocities due to respiration.

Congenital anomalies

CLASSIFICATION

Abnormalities in:

- number (renal agenesis)
- position (ptosis, ectopia)
- fusion (horseshoe, crossed fused ectopia).

Renal agenesis

Early insult to developing ureteral bud – a normal kidney fails to form. It may be detected antenatally.

Bilateral

Incompatible with life. This is often detected antenatally

- no renal tissue identified
- oligohydramnios is present.

Unilateral

Absence of one kidney.

Solitary kidney

- normal in size at birth
- hypertrophy within 6–12 months.

DMSA should be performed to exclude small functional ectopic kidney.

ASSOCIATED ANOMALIES

Vater syndrome

Gynaecological anomalies

Unilateral cryptorchidism.

Renal hypoplasia

A congenitally small kidney is present but with normal architecture.

ULTRASOUND APPEARANCES

Unilateral

- A small kidney, with normal corticomedullary differentiation is noted.
- Compensatory hypertrophy of the contralateral kidney is present.

Bilateral

This is associated with chronic renal failure which becomes clinically apparent at a variable age depending on the severity of the hypoplasia.

- Small kidneys.
- Loss of corticomedullary differentiation.
- The cortex appears 'hyperechoic'.

Renal ectopia

Failure of ascent of the kidneys from the pelvis in utero.

Usually asymptomatic but patients with ectopic kidneys have increased risk of infection and hydronephrosis.

There is often an unusual shape with malrotation and an unusual distribution of the calyces.

The most frequent location of the ectopic kidney is the pelvis.

A rare variant is the thoracic kidney. The kidney migrates upwards and is seen posteriorly under a localised eventration of the diaphragm.

Renal fusion

Horseshoe kidney
Commonest form of fusion (Fig. 11.4).

The lower poles are joined by an isthmus of renal tissue, which lies anterior to the aorta and IVC.

ULTRASOUND APPEARANCES
- Medially orientated lower poles with an isthmus of renal tissue across the midline.
- Bowel gas may prevent ultrasonic visualisation of the isthmus.
- A significant difference in size of the two renal elements is often present. The orientation of the kidneys is variable due to associated malrotation.

Crossed fused ectopia

Both kidneys lie on the same side of the abdomen and are fused. (Fig. 11.5). The ureters enter the bladder in the normal position.

The usual orientation is one above the other, resulting in an S-shape.

ULTRASOUND APPEARANCES
- Absence of one kidney in its normal position.

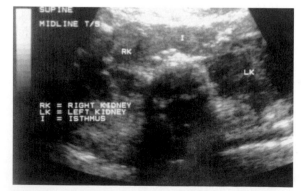

Figure 11.4 — Horseshoe kidney. Typical appearance in transverse section with the isthmus lying anterior to the vertebra.

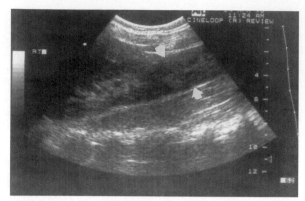

Figure 11.5 — Crossed fused ectopia. The arrows point to the ectopic contralateral kidney.

- A mass with renal contour and two separate renal sinus echoes.

TIPS
If a kidney is not found in its normal location in the loin and the second kidney is normal in size for age, there will almost certainly be an ectopically situated kidney in the abdomen. This can be difficult to identify, but is easily located by radionuclide studies. If the normally positioned kidney is hypertrophied there may or may not be an ectopic kidney. Radionuclide studies with anterior views and masking off of the normal kidney is the best method of locating small renal remnants.

Small ectopically located kidneys may present clinically with constant wetting due to the ureter entering the vagina below the bladder sphincters. A negative ultrasound examination does not exclude such a kidney.

Duplex anomalies

Duplication of the renal collecting system. This is the most common renal anomaly. It may be bilateral or unilateral. The anomaly ranges from partial to complete separation of the collecting system with two ureters entering the bladder. Partial duplication anomaly encompasses a bifid collecting system with a single renal pelvis and ureter to complete renal duplication with the ureters joining anywhere along the course of the ureters.

CLINICAL PRESENTATION
Antenatal.

Abdominal pain with or without urinary tract infection.

An incidental finding on routine ultrasound.

Rarely, a prolapsing ureterocele is seen in the vagina.

Palpable kidneys and bladder if a ureterocele causes bladder outlet obstruction.

ULTRASOUND APPEARANCES

- The kidney is larger than normal.

- Two separate sinus echoes are identifiable (Fig. 11.6).

Complete duplication

The kidney has two completely separate collecting systems, with ureters which insert ectopically into the bladder. The ureter from the upper moiety enters the bladder medially and inferiorly to the lower moiety ureter. The upper moiety ureter may be associated with a ureterocele. The lower moiety ureter inserts laterally and superiorly to its normal position, predisposing to vesico-ureteric reflux, although this is not always present.

ULTRASOUND APPEARANCES

A variety of patterns are seen.

- Variable degree of dilatation of the upper moiety with parenchymal thinning and a tortuous dilated ureter, often with a ureterocele in the bladder (Fig. 11.7a,b).

- Cystic mass at the upper pole, with only a thin rim of cortex. The ureter is usually dilated as above.

- A highly echogenic upper pole; dysplastic or hypoplastic rather than dilated. Ureteric dilatation is variable.

- A dilated ureter, with a ureterocele in the bladder. This is unusual without upper tract dilatation.

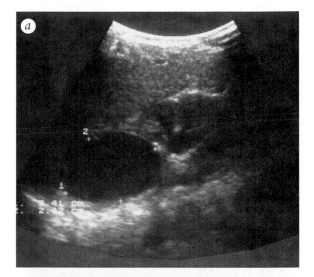

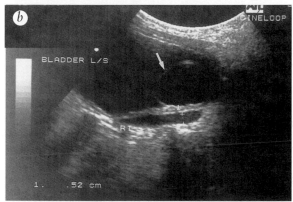

Figure 11.7 — (a) Obstructed upper moiety of a duplex kidney. The anechoic 'mass' is the obstructed upper pole. (b) Same patient. Note the linear anechoic structure which is the dilated ureter behind the bladder and the distended ureterocele within the bladder (arrow).

- Dilatation of the lower moiety ureter due to reflux often accompanied by focal scarring and loss of normal renal volume.

- Dilatation of the lower moiety and thinning of cortex associated with reflux.

FURTHER IMAGING

This is dictated by clinical symptoms and imaging appearances. DMSA scintigraphy is indicated to assess the function of the two poles.

A micturating cystogram may be needed to assess reflux.

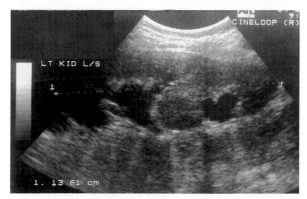

Figure 11.6 — Duplex kidney. Note the two separate renal pelves.

TREATMENT

Surgical management is required and is determined by the degree of upper pole function. If it is non-functioning the usual operation is heminephrectomy. If there is reasonable upper pole function, endoscopic incision of the ureterocele is usually undertaken initially, with further surgery determined by subsequent imaging and symptoms.

Simple ureterocele

There is a small cystic lesion at the insertion of the ureter into the bladder. If this is collapsed it will appear solid. If it contains urine, it will be cystic (Fig. 11.8). The appearance may vary during the examination. A simple ureterocele is not associated with a duplex upper tract.

Hydronephrosis and hydroureteronephrosis

Dilatation of the renal collecting system, which may be confined to the upper tract and is called hydronephrosis; or it may involve both upper tracts and ureter and is hydroureteronephrosis.

CAUSES

The most common include:

Pelviureteric junction (PUJ) obstruction.

Megaureter.

Vesico ureteric obstruction, e.g. calculi, thick walled bladder, or functional.

Isolated upper pole calyceal dilatation.

Megacalycosis (very rare).

Duplex anomalies.

Bladder outlet obstruction, e.g. posterior urethral valves, tumour, prolapsing ureterocele.

Vesico-ureteric reflux, urinary tract infection (UTI).

PUJ obstruction

This is the most common cause of hydronephrosis in the paediatric patient (Fig. 11.9). It is more frequent in boys. It is more frequent on the left. Causes of PUJ obstruction include kinking of the junction, or compression of the junction by a band, adhesion or aberrant vessel, or ureteral stenosis.

CLINICAL PRESENTATION

In the neonate
Antenatal diagnosis.

A palpable mass.

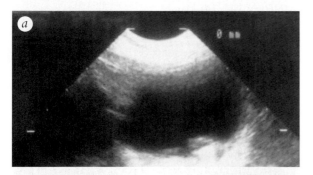
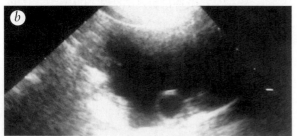

Figure 11.8 — Typical appearance of simple ureterocele within the bladder: (a) collapsed (b) distended.

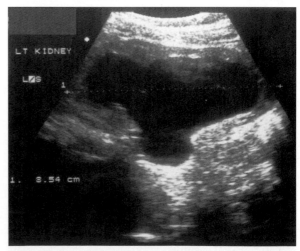

Figure 11.9 — Left kidney with typical configuration of a pelviureteric junction obstruction.

In the older child

Abdominal pain.

Haematuria.

UTI or pyonephrosis.

Palpable mass.

ULTRASOUND APPEARANCES

- Multiple dilated calyces which have a cystic structure of uniform size, communicating with each other and with a medially placed larger 'cyst', the dilated renal pelvis.

- Visible renal cortex which should be assessed for normality of echotexture and have its depth measured.

- No dilatation of the ureter below the renal pelvis.

- Occasionally dilatation of the collecting system of the contralateral kidney due to reflux.

- If infected, the normal anechoic appearance is replaced by echogenic debris which may layer out with positional change.

FURTHER INVESTIGATION

A renogram is required to confirm the US diagnosis and to assess divided renal function.

TREATMENT

Depends on symptoms and renographic results. Surgical pyeloplasty is the usual treatment, when indicated.

Megaureters

These are large dilated ureters with variable degrees of upper tract dilatation. Primary megaureters are usually unilateral.

Primary obstructive megaureter – most frequent

This is a narrowed, distal ureter which is aperistaltic, or will not dilate enough to allow urine to pass through. The narrowing may not be visible on ultrasound. This type is usually associated with upper tract dilatation.

CLINICAL PRESENTATION

Antenatal diagnosis.

UTI.

Haematuria.

Abdominal pain.

ULTRASOUND APPEARANCES

- Tortuous dilated ureters, anechoic tubular structures.

- Narrowing of the distal segment.

- Hyperperistalsis of the ureter proximal to the narrowed distal segment.

Secondary obstructive megaureter

Dilatation of the ureter and usually upper tract as a result of ureteric obstruction at bladder level by calculi (Fig. 11.10), ureterocele (Fig. 11.7b), neurogenic thick walled bladder and, rarely, tumour.

CLINICAL PRESENTATION

Antenatal diagnosis.

UTI.

Haematuria.

Abdominal pain.

ULTRASOUND APPEARANCES

- Tortuous dilated ureters.

- Distal dilated ureter more dilated than the proximal ureter.

- Ureterocele may or may not be present.

- Calculi.

- Neuropathic bladder.

Non-obstructive megaureter

This appears the same as an obstructive megaureter ultrasonically, but has normal drainage at renography and often has normal upper tracts.

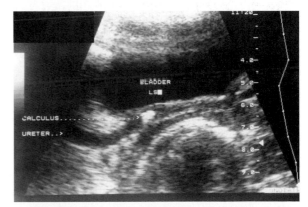

Figure 11.10 — Obstructed ureter behind the bladder, due to a calculus at the vesicoureteric junction.

CLINICAL PRESENTATION

Usually an incidental finding during ultrasound for some other reason. May also be seen with vesico-ureteric reflux.

Vesico-ureteric obstruction

Obstruction at the distal end of the ureter, e.g. calculus (Fig. 11.10), ureterocele (Fig. 11.7b) or neurogenic bladder.

CLINICAL PRESENTATION

Antenatal detection if due to ureterocele.

Urinary tract infection.

Pain.

ULTRASOUND APPEARANCES

- Dilated ureter which may be tortuous.
- Hydroureteronephrosis.
- Associated cause, e.g. ureterocele, calculus.

Neurogenic bladder
The bladder wall is thick. The posterior urethra may be open. There may be bladder wall irregularity, due to multiple diverticulae.

Ureteric stone
This, if impacted in the distal ureter, will cast an acoustic shadow behind it. There are variable degrees of ureteric dilatation (Fig. 11.10).

TREATMENT

Surgical management to relieve the obstruction, pre-serve renal function and prevent infection may be required. Renal function is first assessed by radio-nuclide imaging.

Bladder outlet obstruction

The commonest cause in children is posterior urethral valves. Second most frequent is neurogenic bladder, seen in spina bifida or spinal cord lesions. Rarely, tumours are a cause.

Posterior urethral valves
Congenital valvular obstruction of the posterior male urethra. Early diagnosis is essential to limit damage to renal function.

CLINICAL PRESENTATION

In the neonate
Antenatal diagnosis of a large bladder with hydroureteronephrosis, usually bilateral.

Palpable kidneys and bladder.

Absence of a good urinary stream.

In the older child
UTI.

Palpable kidneys.

Renal failure.

Micturition problems.

ULTRASOUND APPEARANCES
- Bilateral hydronephrosis (Fig. 11.11a).
- Loss of cortical depth; the remaining cortex should be measured.

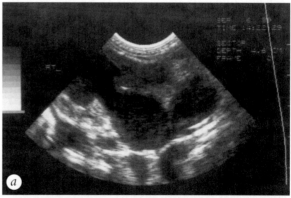

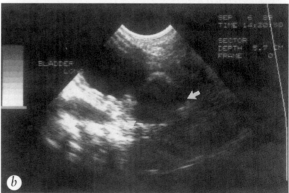

Figure 11.11 — (a) Hydronephrosis secondary to posterior urethral valves causing bladder outlet obstruction. The increased echoes in the renal pelvis are due to infected urine. (b) The bladder wall is thickened and the posterior uretha dilated (arrow).

- Bilateral, dilated, tortuous ureters.

- A thick-walled bladder (Fig. 11.11b).

- A dilated posterior urethra (Fig. 11.11b).

- Ascites (leakage of urine due to extreme pressure only seen in the neonate).

- Urinoma.

- Variable residual volume following micturition.

- The dilated posterior urethra may be seen by scanning the perineum.

A micturating cystourethrogram under antibiotic cover is required to confirm the diagnosis. Renal function is assessed by renography.

PITFALLS

The ureters may be so tortuous that they resemble multiple intra-abdominal cysts. It can be impossible to trace continuity of a single tubular structure.

In a small percentage of cases, massive reflux to one kidney protects the contralateral kidney from damage so that it appears normal. The presence of a normal system on one side does not exclude valves.

TREATMENT

Surgical ablation of the valves is undertaken. Secondary surgery for relief of obstruction or for treatment of reflux may be subsequently needed.

Isolated upper pole calyceal dilatation

Caused by compression of the calyceal infundibulum by an intrarenal aberrant vessel.

CLINICAL PRESENTATION

An incidental finding on routine sonography.

ULTRASOUND APPEARANCE

- Isolated upper pole calyceal dilatation which causes a cystic appearance (Fig. 11.12),

- It may be impossible to trace the connection to the rest of the collecting system; therefore difficult to distinguish from a simple cyst.

- The latter is often more spherical.

FURTHER INVESTIGATIONS

Renography will show retention of isotope in the obstructed calyx.

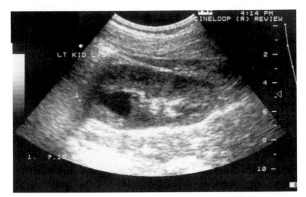

Figure 11.12 — Isolated upper pole calyceal dilatation. The cystic area in the upper pole of the kidney is the dilated calyx.

TREATMENT

None required.

Megacalycosis

Congenital dilatation of and increase in number of the calyces in a kidney without dilatation of the renal pelvis or ureter. This is a rare anomaly.

CLINICAL PRESENTATION

Usually an incidental finding on routine sonography.

ULTRASOUND APPEARANCE

The kidney is usually enlarged with a good cortical depth, variable dilatation of the renal calyces but no renal pelvic dilatation.

FURTHER INVESTIGATION

Renography or an IVU will show the anatomy and demonstrate renal drainage.

TREATMENT

None required.

Urinary tract infections

Urinary tract infection is common in childhood, especially in girls. The purpose of ultrasound is:

To exclude an underlying structural abnormality

To identify renal scars

To measure renal size as a baseline for monitoring growth.

CLINICAL PRESENTATION

Fever.

Abdominal pain.

Haematuria.

Vomiting.

Smelly urine.

Frequency of micturition.

Enuresis.

Failure to thrive.

Vesico-ureteric reflux

This is commonly seen in patients with UTI. There is an increased familial incidence. It is not usually associated with an existing structural abnormality, but can occasionally be seen in the following:

Abnormality of the VUJ.

Neurogenic bladder.

Posterior urethral valves.

Duplex systems.

Megaureters.

ULTRASOUND APPEARANCES

- Normal examination.

- Dilatation of the distal ureters but may be intermittent (Fig. 11.13).

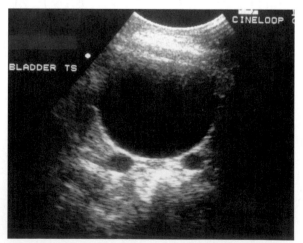

Figure 11.13 — Transverse view of the bladder showing dilated ureters behind it. This was due to vesico-ureteric reflux.

- Scarring, manifested by an irregular renal outline, loss of cortical depth, or altered echopattern in the renal cortex (Fig. 11.14).

- If reflux is severe, small scarred kidneys.

Ultrasound cannot reliably diagnose reflux or renal scarring. An MCU and scintigraphy are required to confirm diagnosis. The role of ultrasound is discussed above. However, normal renal ultrasound diminishes the likelihood of reflux or renal scarring.

TREATMENT

Correction of a structural anomaly may be curative. Most children without a structural abnormality are treated conservatively with antibiotics. Some children require anti–reflux surgery but most will respond to conservative management.

The ureters can be re-implanted; postoperative ultrasound may show localised thickening of the bladder wall. The STING (sub-ureteric Teflon or collagen injection) procedure is also used to prevent reflux. Ultrasound demonstrates an echogenic area with acoustic shadowing at the vesicoureteric junction. (Fig. 11.15).

Acute pyelonephritis

The most common causative organism is *E. coli*.

CLINICAL PRESENTATION

Fever.

Tenderness localised to the kidney area.

Haematuria.

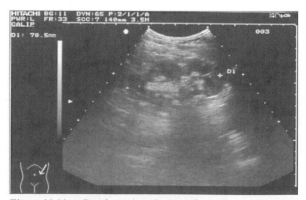

Figure 11.14 — Renal scarring. An irregular outline and marked loss of renal cortex consistent with renal scarring.

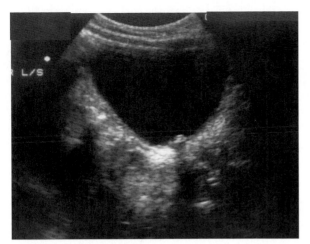

Figure 11.15 — Post 'STING' procedure. The echogenic lesion in the bladder with acoustic shadowing is due to the subureteric Teflon deposition.

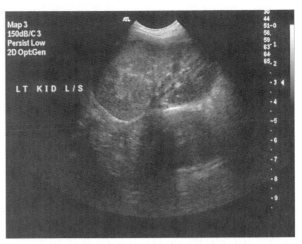

Figure 11.16 — Acute pyelonephritis. Focal enlargement of the upper pole of the left kidney with loss of normal corticomedullary differentiation.

ULTRASOUND APPEARANCES

The appearance is variable:

- Normal appearances and size.

- Increase in kidney size.

- Hypoechoic cortex.

- Loss of corticomedullary differentiation (Fig. 11.16).

- Focal infection, a hypoechoic area within the kidney.

FURTHER INVESTIGATION

Follow up ultrasound and scintigraphy to establish the presence of renal damage.

TREATMENT
Antibiotics.

Chronic pyelonephritis (Reflux nephropathy)

Repeated infections destroy the kidneys.

ULTRASOUND APPEARANCES

- Small kidneys.

- Echogenic with an irregular outline due to scarring.

- Loss of corticomedullary differentiation.

- Dilatation of the collecting system.

FURTHER INVESTIGATION

Scintigraphy to establish divided renal function.

TREATMENT

Antibiotics and treatment of renal failure, as indicated.

Renal abscess

Failure of treatment in acute pyelonephritis or haematogenous dissemination of a distant infection may result in a renal abscess (Fig. 11.17).

CLINICAL PRESENTATION

Fever and loin pain.

Pyuria or haematuria may be present.

ULTRASOUND APPEARANCES

- Variable.

- Well-defined mass.

- Irregular or well defined thick walls.

- Anechoic mass with cystic enhancement.

- Internal echoes, depending on the amount of debris within the abscess.

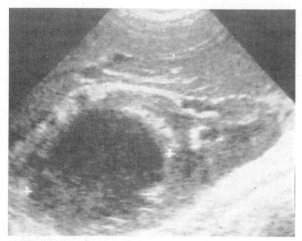

Figure 11.17 — Large renal abscess. Note the hypoechoic mass lesion distorting the upper pole outline.

- Bright echoes with shadowing representing gas-forming organisms.
- Fluid/debris level.

FURTHER INVESTIGATION
CT may be required to image the full extent.

TREATMENT
Intravenous antibiotics and, when indicated, drainage. Renal damage is monitored by scintigraphy.

Pyonephrosis

Pus in a dilated collecting system, often secondary to a congenital anomaly, e.g. PUJ obstruction, but may be due to a calculus or stricture.

CLINICAL PRESENTATION
Fever and loin pain.

Pyuria is common.

ULTRASOUND APPEARANCES
- Dilated collecting system containing debris (Fig. 11.18).
- Fluid/fluid or fluid/debris levels, which change with patient position.
- Bright echoes with shadowing representing gas forming organisms.

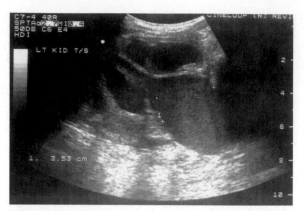

Figure 11.18 — Typical appearance of pyonephrosis. The dilated collecting system contains echogenic urine.

FURTHER INVESTIGATION
Monitoring of resolution of the pyonephrosis is by ultrasound. Once the child recovers, renal function is assessed by scintigraphy.

TREATMENT
Acute management: antibiotics and percutaneous drainage of the system. Further surgery may be required to treat the primary lesions.

Fungal balls

Result from fungal infection of the kidney. The most common causative agent is *Candida albicans*.

This is more common in:

Immunocompromised patients.

Premature infants.

Patients with indwelling catheters.

CLINICAL PRESENTATION
Fever.

Pain if there is obstruction caused by the fungal ball.

ULTRASOUND APPEARANCES
- Echogenic masses within the collecting system of the kidney (Fig. 11.19).
- Lack of acoustic shadowing; differentiates this from calculi.
- Hydronephrosis with debris.

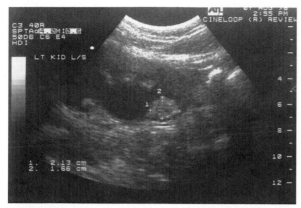

Figure 11.19 — Fungus balls in the collecting system. The echogenic lesions typically fill the calyx but do not demonstrate acoustic shadowing.

FURTHER INVESTIGATION

Monitoring of progress of treatment by serial ultrasound.

Scintigraphy to assess function.

TREATMENT

Antifungal agents. Obstruction may need to be relieved by percutaneous drainage.

Xanthogranulomatous pyelonephritis

A particular form of chronic renal abscess in which there is an abdominal mass which contains calcification and areas of fatty infiltration due to the xanthogranulomatous tissue. It may arise in a normal kidney or be a complication of infection in a hydronephrotic kidney.

CLINICAL PRESENTATION

Pain.

Palpable abdominal mass.

Fever, often low grade.

Chronic ill health.

ULTRASOUND APPEARANCE

A large irregular loin mass of mixed echo pattern, containing areas of calcification with acoustic shadowing and areas of increased echogenicity due to the xanthogranulomatous material (Fig. 11.20).

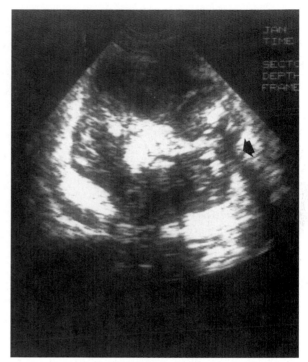

Figure 11.20 — Xanthogranulomatous pyelonephritis. Note the irregular renal outline with a mixed echo pattern and some acoustic shadowing (arrow). This is due to calcification. The bright echoes represent fat.

TREATMENT

Nephrectomy and antibiotics.

Urolithiasis

The presence of calculi within the renal tract.

Less common in children than adults.

CAUSES

Infection.

Metabolic abnormalities.

CLINICAL PRESENTATION

UTI.

Haematuria.

Abdominal pain.

Painful micturition.

ULTRASOUND APPEARANCES

- A highly echogenic focus which, depending on its size, may or may not cast an acoustic shadow. If it is seen within the collecting system. It may or may not be accompanied by dilatation (Fig. 11.21).

- Stones in the distal ureter are usually associated with proximal obstructive hydronephrosis (see Fig. 11.10).

- Stones located in the distal ureter may be missed if the bladder is not full.

- Stones located in the mid ureter may be difficult to identify due to interference from abdominal gas but, if there is proximal obstruction, the dilatation is visible.

- Associated signs e.g. hydronephrosis.

PITFALL

- In the neonate, fungus balls due to candida septicaemia appear as echogenic foci in the calyces but do not cast an acoustic shadow (Fig. 11.19).

Nephrocalcinosis

The localised or diffuse deposition of calcium in the renal parenchyma – bilateral.

CAUSES

In neonates and infants

Frusemide therapy.

Frusemide inhibits calcium reabsorption causing hypercalcaemia.

Renal tubular acidosis (Fig. 11.22).

Bartters and Williams syndrome.

Metabolic disorders.

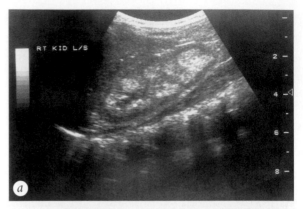

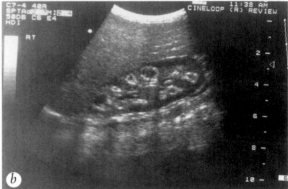

Figure 11.22 — (a & b) Nephrocalcinosis. The bright symmetrically arranged echoes are due to calcium deposition within the renal tubules. Two patterns are illustrated.

In older children

Renal tubular acidosis

Metabolic disorders

Medullary sponge kidneys

Various syndromes.

Nephrocalcinosis usually affects both kidneys, but can be unilateral.

Ultrasound appearances

DIFFUSE DISEASE:

Generalised increased echogenicity of the parenchyma.

Localised to medullary area:

Echogenic pyramids – Anderson-Carr progression – initially seen in the tip of the pyramid and then throughout the pyramid.

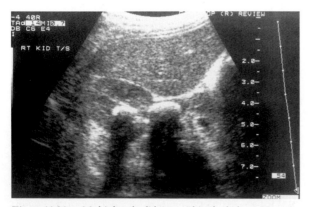

Figure 11.21 — Multiple calculi lying within the kidney. Note the acoustic shadowing cast by these.

- Reversed cortico-medullary differentiation.
- Depending on the size of calcification, there may or may not be acoustic shadowing.
- The kidney may be more echogenic than the liver or spleen.

Renal cystic disease

Simple cysts

Rare in children. Usually single, occasionally multiple.

Known syndromes associated with simple cortical cysts: e.g. Tuberous sclerosis

Zellweger's

Von Hippel-Lindau

Down's

Turner's.

CLINICAL PRESENTATION

Usually asymptomatic. If they are large or have had haemorrhage into them, they may present with pain.

ULTRASOUND APPEARANCES

- Spherical or oval anechoic lesions (Fig. 11.23).
- Thin-walled.
- Contain no internal echoes, unless complicated by haemorrhage or infection.

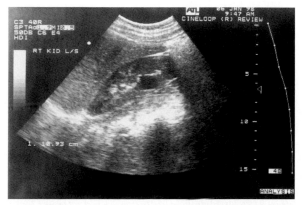

Figure 11.23 — Simple renal cyst. Typical appearance of an anechoic lesion which may be located anywhere in the kidney.

- Demonstrate acoustic enhancement.
- Are not in communication with the collecting system.

Autosomal recessive polycystic disease

(Infantile polycystic disease)

Congenital. Inherited as a recessive characteristic but with variable expression of severity.

Bilateral.

Numerous small cysts within the cortex and medulla.

Associated with hepatic fibrosis.

CLINICAL PRESENTATION

Neonatal period
Bilateral enlarged kidneys

Decreased renal function

Often detected antenatally.

Childhood
Hepatic disease dominates

Presentation is usually with portal hypertension

Milder involvement of the kidneys compared to the neonate.

ULTRASOUND APPEARANCES

Neonates
Bilaterally enlarged kidneys > 8 cm.

- Diffusely echogenic (Fig. 11.24).
- Loss of cortico-medullary differentiation.
- A hypoechoic subcapsular rim is often visible.
- Normal or slightly bright liver (minimal fibrosis).

Older children
- Diffusely echogenic kidneys (Fig. 11.25).
- Prominent pyramids/hyperechoic cortex.
- The liver appears 'bright' if there is periportal fibrosis.
- Splenomegaly due to portal hypertension is common.
- Doppler studies may show evidence of portal hypertension.

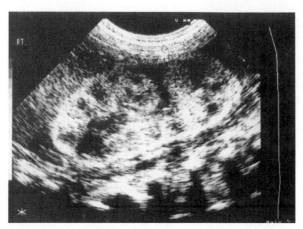

Figure 11.24 — Patient with typical appearances of infantile polycystic disease. Note complete loss of normal structure of the kidney, which is echogenic.

Autosomal dominant polycystic kidney disease

(Adult polycystic disease)

Familial.

Bilateral involvement of the kidneys but often one side is more affected initially.

Associated with liver and pancreatic cysts progressively appearing with age.

Usually > 20 years, but increasingly being seen in children because of family screening.

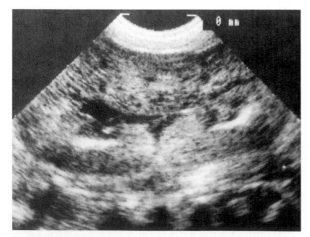

Figure 11.25 — Patient who presented at age 8 with an enlarged liver. Note echogenic kidney which is due to the polycystic kidney associated with hepatic fibrosis.

CLINICAL PRESENTATION

Haematuria.

Hypertension.

Detection because of familial screening.

ULTRASOUND APPEARANCES

- Enlarged kidneys (Fig. 11.26).
- Multiple cysts of varying size.
- Cysts in the liver and pancreas.

Multicystic dysplastic kidney

The second most common cause of an abdominal mass in the newborn (the first is hydronephrosis).

Frequently detected antenatally.

Is secondary to ureteric obstruction early in fetal life.

Has an associated atretic ureter.

Can be associated with an abnormality of the contralateral kidney, e.g. reflux, PUJ.

The kidney is non functioning.

Usually not removed as it involutes spontaneously.

If bilateral, fatal.

ULTRASOUND APPEARANCES

- Anechoic masses of varying size and shape (Fig. 11.27).
- The cysts do not communicate.
- No identifiable renal pelvis.
- No visible renal cortex.

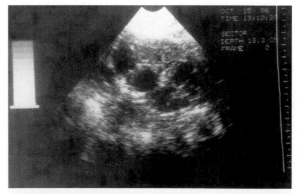

Figure 11.26 — Adult polycystic kidney in a child aged 12 who presented with headache due to hypertension. Note the cystic areas within the kidney.

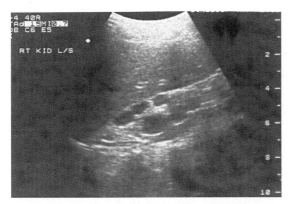

Figure 11.27 — Multicystic dysplastic kidney. Multiple cysts are demonstrated, the renal cortex appears echogenic

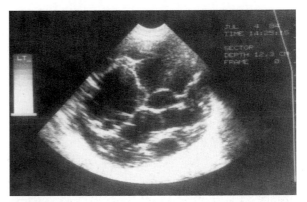

Figure 11.28 — Typical appearance of multilocular cystic nephroma. Note the multiple cysts with septae.

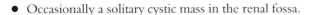

- Occasionally a solitary cystic mass in the renal fossa.
- Hypertrophy of the contralateral kidney.

Multilocular cystic nephroma

Rare.

Non-hereditary.

Affects children < 4 years.

More common in boys.

CLINICAL PRESENTATION

Non painful palpable abdominal mass.

Haematuria.

ULTRASOUND APPEARANCES

- Well defined anechoic mass with septations (Fig. 11.28).
- May or may not involve the whole kidney.
- Easily confused with a cystic Wilms' tumour.

Malignant renal tumours

Wilms' tumour

Most common renal tumour in children.

Usually occurs before 5 years of age.

Can be unilateral or bilateral.

ASSOCIATED ANOMALIES

Hemi-hypertrophy

Beckwith-Weidemann syndrome

Aniridia

Nephroblastomatosis.

CLINICAL PRESENTATION

Asymptomatic rapidly growing abdominal mass.

Pain.

Haematuria (microscopic).

Fever.

Hypertension.

ULTRASOUND APPEARANCES

- Well defined, large, mainly solid mass (Fig. 11.29).
- Heterogeneous or homogeneous texture.
- Echogenicity similar to or slightly less than the liver.
- Anechoic areas, representing necrosis or haemorrhage (Fig. 11.30)
- Bright areas which are usually haemorrhagic necrosis.
- Calcification is uncommon but does rarely occur. If seen consider neuroblastoma.
- Displacement of local structures, e.g. liver, IVC.
- Enlarged nodes, not always visible even when present. May be obscured due to large mass.
- Extension to involve the renal vein or IVC with tumour thrombus in the lumen (Fig. 11.31). Failure

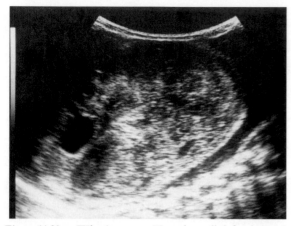

Figure 11.29 — Wilms' tumour. Note the well defined mass in the kidney with loss of the normal architecture. The hypoechoic rim around the kidney is due to a perirenal fluid collection of blood.

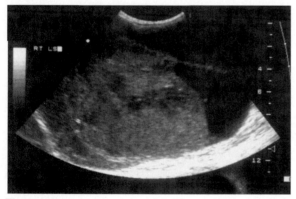

Figure 11.30 — Large mainly solid Wilms' with anechoic areas representing necrosis.

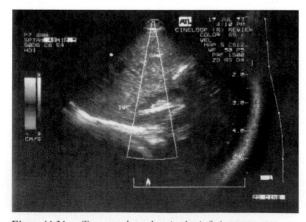

Figure 11.31 — Tumour thrombus in the inferior vena cava.

to show IVC may be due to compression and not tumour thrombus.

- Free fluid if there is capsular rupture.

- Some normal renal tissue around the mass is usually detectable.

- Metastases in the liver appear hypoechoic.

- Always look carefully for involvement of the contralateral kidney.

STAGING OF A WILMS' TUMOUR

Stage 1 – Well defined tumour. No spread.

Stage 2 – Local infiltration beyond the capsule

Stage 3 – Local extension beyond the kidney
– Spread to the peritoneum
– Enlarged nodes

Stage 4 – Metastases, e.g. liver, lung

Stage 5 – Bilateral renal involvement

Renal cell carcinoma

Rare in childhood; usually mistaken for a Wilms'.

Peak age of incidence is 9 years.

Cannot be distinguished from a Wilms' tumour by imaging.

Poor prognosis.

Metastasises to both liver and lungs.

CLINICAL PRESENTATION

Abdominal mass.

Pain.

Haematuria (frank).

ULTRASOUND APPEARANCES

- Variable.

- Homogeneous/heterogeneous solid renal mass.

- Size variable.

- Calcification commoner than with Wilms'.

- Evidence of spread to involve retroperitoneum.

- Lymph nodes and renal vein.

Lymphoma

Primary lymphoma is rare.

Metastatic involvement occurs in Stage 4 disease, with disease evident elsewhere.

Most commonly seen in:

Non-Hodgkin's lymphoma

B-cell Burkitt lymphoma.

ULTRASOUND APPEARANCES
- Renal enlargement, usually bilateral (Fig. 11.32).
- Discrete renal masses which appear anechoic or hypoechoic but without acoustic enhancement.
- Diffuse infiltration; the kidney appears hypoechoic.

Leukaemia

Acute leukaemia is the most common malignancy in children.

Peak age of incidence is 3–5 years.

Kidney involvement is not infrequent at presentation.

CLINICAL PRESENTATION
Leukaemia involvement of the kidney rarely presents clinically, but can result in:

Abdominal pain.

Haematuria.

Hypertension.

Renal failure.

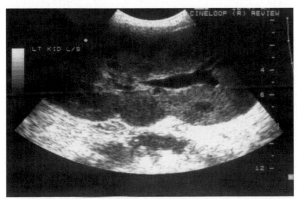

Figure 11.32 — Lymphoma within the kidney. The kidney is enlarged and has a lobulated outline due to the lymphomatous deposit.

ULTRASOUND APPEARANCES
- Symmetrical, bilateral nephromegaly.
- Smooth outline.
- Normal to slightly increased echogenicity.
- Loss of cortico-medullary differentiation.
- Hydronephrosis: pressure effect if there are enlarged retroperitoneal nodes.

Benign renal tumours

Angiomyolipoma

Rare.

Associated with tuberous sclerosis.

Uncommon in childhood.

CLINICAL PRESENTATION
Small lesions – asymptomatic.

Extensive involvement – renal failure.

ULTRASOUND APPEARANCES
- Small echogenic areas, representing fat, therefore no acoustic shadowing.
- Diffuse increase in echogenicity as a result of near total replacement of the kidney by angiomyolipomas.

Mesoblastic nephroma

(Congenital Wilms' tumour)

Most common tumour in children < 1 year.

May be detected antenatally.

CLINICAL PRESENTATION
Painless abdominal mass.

Occasionally hypertension.

ULTRASOUND APPEARANCES
- Large well defined homogeneous mass (Fig. 11.33).
- Sometimes contains irregular anechoic areas representing necrosis or haemorrhage.

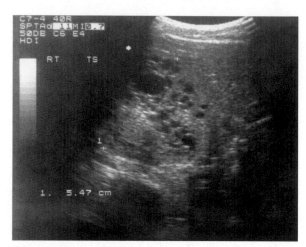

Figure 11.33 — Mesoblastic nephroma. Note the relatively homogeneous mass with anechoic areas representing necrosis.

TREATMENT

Removal.

Chemotherapy is not necessary.

Renal trauma

The kidney is less commonly injured than the liver and spleen in blunt abdominal trauma but a congenitally abnormal kidney is more easily injured than a normal kidney. The main cause is road traffic accidents or hyperflexion falls. It can result from a renal biopsy, but usually only small lacerations or haematomas are seen. CT is the investigation of choice for full demonstration of the lesion, with radionuclide studies for functional assessment. Ultrasound is useful in demonstrating haematomas and contusions, the integrity of main vessels and traumatic urinomas. Monitoring of resolution of the injury and long-term damage to the kidney is best achieved by ultrasound.

CLINICAL PRESENTATION

Macroscopic haematuria.

Blunt abdominal trauma

ULTRASOUND APPEARANCES

These are variable and depend on the severity of trauma.

- Haematomas
    - mass with irregular walls.
    - appearance depends on its age.
    - as organisation occurs contains internal echoes.
    - as resolution occurs appears more hypo/anechoic.
- Lacerations
    - linear hypo/hyperechoic defects.
    - abnormality of the renal outline (Fig. 11.34).
- Perirenal/Subcapsular haematomas
    - complex crescent-shaped hyper/hypoechoic fluid collection.
- Contusions
    - areas of increased echogenicity initially progressing to liquefaction and fibrosis.
- Urinoma
    - normally hypoechoic but if mixed blood and urine will have a mixed echotexture (Fig. 11.35).

Renal vein thrombosis

Usually occurs in the neonate.

More common in infants of diabetic mothers.

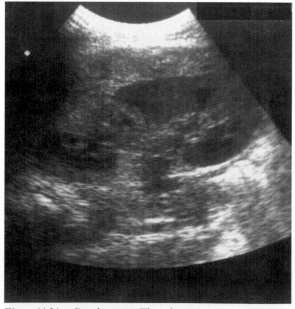

Figure 11.34 — Renal trauma. The echogenic region in the upper pole is due to an area of contusion.

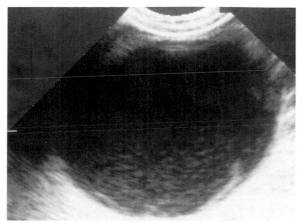

Figure 11.35 — Large urinoma containing echogenic debris.

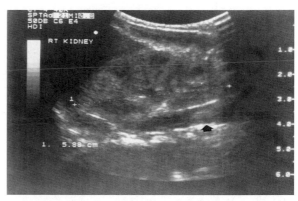

Figure 11.36 — Renal vein thrombosis. The right kidney is enlarged with loss of the normal architecture and is more hyperechoic than normal. Thrombus (arrow) is present within the IVC.

CLINICAL PRESENTATION

Dehydration due to blood loss, sepsis, diarrhoea.

Renal insufficiency.

Painful flank mass.

Haematuria.

Transient hypertension.

Can be asymptomatic.

Has been described antenatally.

ULTRASOUND APPEARANCES

- Variable.
- Hyperechoic perilobar and interlobar streaks are seen in both acute and chronic renal vein thrombosis (Fig. 11.36).
- Thrombus in the IVC (Fig. 11.36).
- Absence of flow in the renal vein on Doppler imaging

In the acute phase
- Enlarged kidney.
- Loss of cortico-medullary differentiation.

NB. These changes are reversible and follow-up ultrasound is usually normal.

In the chronic stage
- Hyperechoic streaks around the pyramids representing calcification secondary to haemorrhage.
- Small kidney with normal cortico-medullary differentiation.

NB. These are permanent changes.

ASSOCIATIONS

Adrenal haemorrhage.

Renal artery thrombosis

Rare, less common than renal vein thrombosis. Increased incidence in infants of diabetic mothers.

CLINICAL PRESENTATION

Sepsis.

Dehydration.

Haemoconcentration.

Patients with indwelling, umbilical artery catheters.

ULTRASOUND APPEARANCES

Acute

- Normal in size with increased echogenicity.
- Thrombus in the renal artery.
- Absence of Doppler signal in the renal artery.

The end result depends on the extent of the insult – small echogenic kidney.

Haemolytic uraemic syndrome

Usually occurs in children younger than 5 years.

Thought to be due to an antibody–antigen reaction to bacterial toxins.

CLINICAL PRESENTATION

Gastroenteritis (bloody).

Thrombocytopenia.

Renal failure.

Hypertension.

ULTRASOUND APPEARANCES

- Mild: normal appearances.

- Severe: increased echogenicity of the cortex, but cortico-medullary differentiation is maintained (Fig. 11.37).

As the patient clinically returns to normal, so do the ultrasound appearances of the kidneys, but dialysis may be required during recovery.

End stage kidney

The common pathway of a variety of renal diseases is that the kidney becomes small, loses all architecture and is hyperechoic (Fig. 11.38).

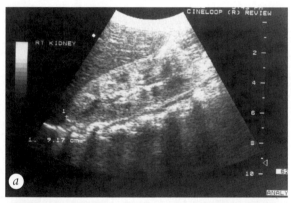

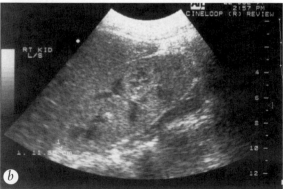

Figure 11.37 — Haemolytic uraemic syndrome. The kidney is hyperechoic relative to the liver. Two patients (a & b) are shown at different stages of evolution.

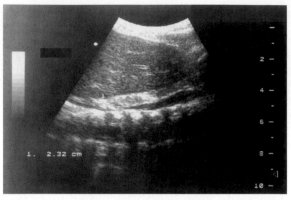

Figure 11.38 — End stage kidney. Note the small hyperechoic kidney with complete loss of architecture. This can be the end result of a variety of causes.

Renal artery stenosis

Rarely visible with ultrasound, but Doppler studies may demonstrate evidence of narrowing. The stenotic site is usually at the junction of the aorta and renal artery which is often difficult to visualise due to overlying bowel gas. Doppler demonstrates increased peak frequency shift at the stenotic site with turbulence and damping of signal distal to the stenosis.

Renal transplant

LOCATION

The patient's pelvis.

APPEARANCE

Should have the same appearance as a normal kidney.

ROUTINE SURVEILLANCE

Renal ultrasound to confirm normal appearance of kidney.

Doppler ultrasound of renal artery and vein to confirm normal flow.

ULTRASOUND APPEARANCES OF COMPLICATIONS

Acute rejection

- Loss of normal echogenic pattern of the kidney with loss of cortico-medullary differentiation.

- Doppler shows diminished forward flow in diastole with increased resistive index (RI).

Renal artery or vein thrombosis

- Loss of normal Doppler flow signal in the vessel.

Urological complications

- Hydronephrosis: caused by ischaemia or oedema of the anastomosis. Follow-up scans with resolution indicate oedema.

- Urinomas: caused by an anastomotic leak. A sonolucent clear perirenal collection is seen. If infected, echoes and debris are seen within the collection

- Lymphocele: seen as a local transonic fluid collection (Fig. 11.39).

Late complications

- Rejection: similar appearances as in the acute phase.

- Cyclosporin toxicity: alteration in echogenic pattern, loss of cortico-medullary differentiation. Reduced flow on Doppler. Biopsy is required to distinguish rejection and cyclosporin toxicity.

- Renal artery stenosis: can cause reduced renal function and hypertension.
  Doppler studies of the vessel show altered waveform, and increased RI.

- Hydronephrosis: late onset hydronephrosis may reflect fibrosis and ischaemia at the anastomosis.

URINARY BLADDER

Normal appearances

A transonic structure variable in size and shape. It is smooth in outline with a mildly echogenic wall, less than 3 mm in thickness when adequately distended (Fig. 11.40).

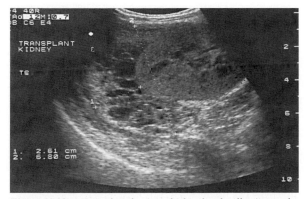

Figure 11.39 — Lymphocele. A multi-loculated collection at the lower pole of the transplant kidney.

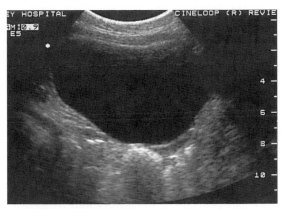

Figure 11.40 — Normal bladder. Ultrasound appearances of the normal bladder in longitudinal section.

In transverse section the bladder demonstrates indentations on its lateral walls, to help identify it from other cystic masses in the pelvis.

The distal ureters are sometimes visualised behind the bladder; less than 2 mm in diameter is considered normal. It is important to watch the ureter peristalsing as this will help to discriminate between ureters and blood vessels.

Congenital anomalies

Agenesis

Very rare. Seen in stillborn infants and usually associated with other anomalies.

Cloacal anomalies

The intestinal, genital and urinary tract are connected and there is a single perineal orifice.

Persistent urogenital sinus

The vagina and urethra are joined. The urethral orifice opens into the anterior wall of the vagina. Reflux is a common problem.

Bladder exstrophy

The bladder is located outside the abdomen. The upper tracts are usually normal at birth, but after bladder reconstruction frequent follow-up is required to assess for possible hydronephrosis.

Epispadias

Abnormal dorsal opening of the male urethra. These children often have a poorly developed bladder neck, and are therefore incontinent of urine.

The role of ultrasound in these conditions is to identify the upper renal tract, and to assess any associated dilatation, and to monitor progress. In females with cloacal anomalies or urogenital sinus anomalies, ultrasound is used in addition to identify the uterus, vagina and ovaries.

Urachal anomalies

The urachus is the allantoic remnant between the umbilicus and the dome of the bladder.

There are four types of anomaly:

Completely patent

Seen as a tubular structure which joins the umbilicus to the superior aspect of the bladder; it can be partially cystic.

Urachal sinus

(Opens to the umbilicus). A cystic tubular structure which communicates with the umbilicus.

Urachal diverticulum

(Opens to the bladder). Can be seen with ultrasound at the superior aspect of the bladder as a cystic area. An MCU would be the examination of choice.

Urachal cysts

A mass found between umbilicus and the dome of the bladder. They are typically cystic, but may be echogenic when infected (Fig. 11.41).

Large bladders

Easily assessed with ultrasound. The bladder extends above the umbilicus and does not empty.

Results from:

Bladder outlet obstruction

Neurogenic abnormalities both occult and obvious

Gross reflux.

Enuresis

May be both diurnal and nocturnal. Usually no associated renal or neurogenic anomaly. Role of ultrasound is to:

Exclude anomaly.

Assess bladder volume both pre and post micturition.

Neuropathic bladder

Neurological conditions which affect the bladder are usually congenital, e.g.

myelomeningocele

sacral agenesis

Acquired forms include:

cerebral palsy

trauma resulting from para/quadriplegia

infection, e.g. meningitis

tumours of the spinal cord.

ULTRASOUND APPEARANCES

Variable

- Thick walled (Fig. 11.42a).

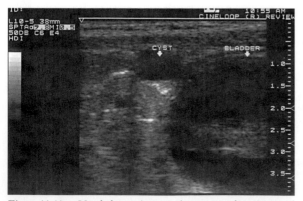

Figure 11.41 — Urachal cyst. A cyst is demonstrated superior and separate from the dome of the bladder.

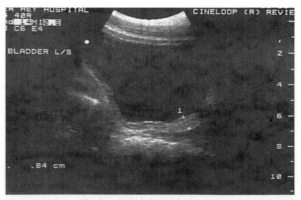

Figure 11.42a — Thick walled bladder. The bladder wall is thickened measuring 8 mm. The normal bladder wall is usually < 3mm.

- Trabeculation (Fig. 11.42b).

- Large post-micturition residue.

- Sometimes dilated upper tracts.

- Echoes within due to infection and debris.

Bladder augmentation

This is required in patients who need urinary tract diversion or reconstruction, i.e. those with small non-compliant bladders, e.g. bladder exstrophy, neuropathic bladders. Ileum, colon or even stomach can be used to make the bladder larger.

ULTRASOUND APPEARANCES

- Irregular shape.

- Debris often seen due to mucus which is secreted by the bowel (Fig. 11.43).

Bladder diverticula

Weakness in the detrusor muscle of the bladder wall, through which the bladder mucosa bulges resulting in pouch.

May be congenital or acquired.

Congenital

Tend to be isolated, and often large, in an otherwise normal bladder (Fig. 11.44).

Acquired

Associated with reflux or neuropathic bladders. Multiple diverticula are often seen when the wall is trabeculated.

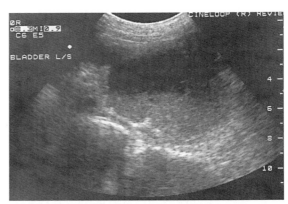

Figure 11.43 — Bladder augmentation. The bladder is irregular in shape with a trabeculated wall and debris caused by mucus secreted by the bowel which has been used to make the bladder larger.

ULTRASOUND APPEARANCES

- Anechoic fluid collection projecting from the bladder wall.

- Smooth bladder wall/trabeculated bladder wall.

Infection

Can cause inflammation of the bladder wall. It is usually bacterial in origin (*E. coli*).

CLINICAL PRESENTATION

Dysuria.

Haematuria.

Patients having chemotherapy.

Patients with indwelling catheters.

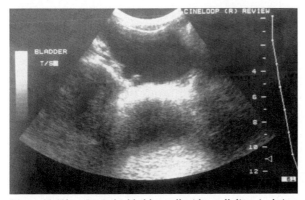

Figure 11.42b — Irregular bladder wall with small diverticula in a patient with myelomeningocele.

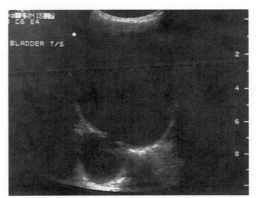

Figure 11.44 — Bladder diverticula. A longitudinal section of the bladder with a smooth walled diverticulum seen posteriorly.

- Uniform or focal bladder wall thickening.
- Debris within the bladder (Fig. 11.45).

NB. Focal bladder wall thickening can also be seen in intra-abdominal inflammatory processes, e.g. perforated appendix, gastroenteritis.

Bladder calculi

Rare, usually from the upper tracts, but can sometimes form in the bladder secondary to infection.

ULTRASOUND APPEARANCES

An echogenic focus with acoustic shadowing, which can be shown to move with patient position (Fig. 11.46).

Bladder injury

In children, the bladder occupies a more abdominal position than in an adult and is therefore more vulnerable to injury.

CLINICAL PRESENTATION

Blunt abdominal trauma.

Previous surgery.

Penetrating injury (e.g. in child abuse).

ULTRASOUND APPEARANCES

- Free fluid
- Defect in the bladder wall

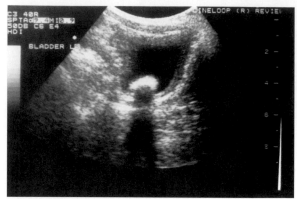

Figure 11.46 — Bladder calculus. Note calculus in the base of the bladder with acoustic shadowing.

Bladder tumour

Uncommon and usually malignant. Rhabdomyosarcoma is the most common. Affects boys more than girls usually below 4 years of age.

CLINICAL PRESENTATION

Abdominal mass.

Haematuria.

Acute urinary retention.

ULTRASOUND APPEARANCES

- A large, lobulated solid mass within the bladder (Fig. 11.47).
- Homogeneous.
- May lie posterior to the bladder and displace it anteriorly.

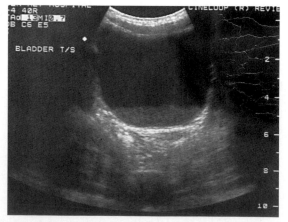

Figure 11.45 — Debris in the bladder. Debris is seen within the bladder in a patient with UTI.

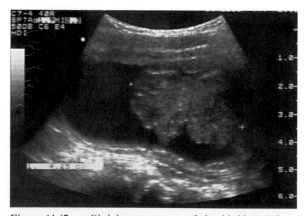

Figure 11.47 — Rhabdomyosarcoma of the bladder. A large lobulated hyperechoic mass is demonstrated within the lumen of the bladder

- Look for secondary features due to compression of ureters or extension to involve them, causing hydronephrosis and dilatation of the ureters proximal to the obstruction.

- Look for pelvic and abdominal nodal disease, and liver metastases, although these are usually to the lung.

TREATMENT

Chemotherapy and surgery.

Frequent follow-up imaging is required to assess shrinkage and recurrence.

Surgical procedures

Mitrofanoff – appendicovesicostomy

The appendix is used to connect the bladder to the skin surface, allowing bladder catheterisation, in patients with chronic outlet obstruction, and those with neuropathic bladders.

Artificial sphincters

Used in patients with neurogenic bladders, an artificial sphincter is put at the bladder neck. The reservoir is seen as a cystic area approximately the size of a 50p coin.

STING – subureteric injection of Teflon

Used in the treatment of reflux. An echogenic focus is seen as the ureter enters the bladder, and causes acoustic shadowing.

Further reading

Ben-Ami T. The sonographic evaluation of urinary tract infections in children. *Semin Ultrasound CT MR* 1984; **5**: 19–34.

Berdon WE, Baker DH, Wigger HJ, Blanc WA. The radiologic and pathologic spectrum of the prune belly syndrome. *Radiol Clin North Am* 1977; **15**: 83–92.

Bis KG, Slovis TL. Accuracy of ultrasonic bladder volume measurement in children. *Pediatr Radiol* 1990 **20**: 457–460.

Blane CE, Barr M, DiPietro MA, Sedman AB, Bloom DA. Renal obstructive dysplasia: ultrasound diagnosis and therapeutic implications. *Pediatr Radiol* 1991; **21**: 274–277.

Blane CE, Bookstein FL, DiPietro MA, Kelsch RC. Sonographic standards for normal infant kidney length. *AJR* 1985; **145**: 1289–1291.

Boal DK, Teele RL. Sonography of infantile polycystic kidney disease. *AJR* 1980; **135**: 575–580.

Brown T, Mandell J, Lebowitz RL. Neonatal hydronephrosis in the era of sonography. *AJR* 1987; **148**: 959–963.

Cacciarelli AA, Kass EJ, Yang SS. Urachal remnants: sonographic demonstration in children. *Radiology* 1990; **174**: 473–475.

Carlson DH, Carlson D, Simon H. Benign multilocular cystic nephroma. *AJR* 1978; **131**: 621–625.

Chan HSL, Cheng M-Y, Mancer K, et al. Congenital mesoblastic nephroma: a clinicoradiologic study of 17 cases representing the pathologic spectrum of the disease. *J Pediatr* 1987; **111**: 64–70.

Choyke PL, Grant EG, Hoffer FA, Tina L, Korec S. Cortical echogenicity in the hemolytic uremic syndrome: clinical correlation. *J Ultrasound Med* 1988; **7**: 439–442.

Cohen HL, Haller JO, Schechter S, Slovis T, Merola R, Eaton DH. Renal candidiasis of the infant: ultrasound evaluation. *Urol Radiol* 1986; **8**: 17–21.

Cohen HL, Susman M, Haller JO, et al. Posterior urethral valve: transperineal US for imaging and diagnosis in male infants. *Radiol* 1994; **192**: 261–264.

Cramer BC, Jequier S, de Chadarevian JP. Factors associated with renal parenchymal echogenicity in the newborn. *J Ultrasound Med* 1986; **5**: 633–638.

Cremin BJ. A review of the ultrasonic appearances of posterior urethral valve and ureteroceles. *Pediatr Radiol* 1986; **16**: 357–364.

Currarino G, Williams B, Dana K. Kidney length correlated with age: normal values in children. *Radiol* 1984; **150**: 703–704.

Davey MS, Zerin JM, Reilly C, Ambrosius WT. Mild renal pelvic dilatation is not predictive of vesicoureteral reflux in children. *Pediatr Radiol* 1997; **27**: 908–911.

Dinkel E, Orth S, Dittrich M, Schulte-Wissermann H. Renal sonography in the differentiation of upper from lower urinary tract infection. *AJR* 1986; **146**: 775–780.

Dodd GD III, Tublin ME, Shah A, Zajko AB. Imaging of vascular complications associated with renal transplants. *AJR* 1991; **157**: 449–459.

Erasmie U, Lidefelt KJ. Accuracy of ultrasonic assessment of residual urine in children. *Pediatr Radiol* 1989; **19**: 388–390.

Fernbach SK, Feinstein KA. Abnormalities of the bladder in children: imaging findings. *AJR* 1994; **162**: 1143–1150.

Fernbach SK, Feinstein KA, Donaldson JS, Baum ES. Nephroblastomatosis: comparison of CT with US and urography. *Radiol* 1988; **166**: 153–156.

Fredericks BJ, de Campo M, Chow CW, Powell HR. Glomerulo-cystic renal disease: ultrasound appearances. *Pediatr Radiol* 1989; **19**: 184–186.

Furtschegger A, Egender G, Jakse G. The value of sonography in the diagnosis and follow-up of patients with blunt renal trauma. *Br J Urol* 1988; **62**: 110–116.

Giuliano CT, Cohen HL, Haller JO, Glassberg KI. The sting procedure and its complications: sonographic evaluation. *J Clin Ultrasound* 1990; **18**: 415–420.

Grossman H, Rosenberg ER, Bowie JD, Ram P, Merten DF. Sonographic diagnosis of renal cystic diseases. *AJR* 1983; **140**: 81–85.

Haller JO, Berdon WE, Friedman AP. Increased renal cortical echogenicity: a normal finding in neonates and infants. *Radiol* 1982; **142**: 173–174.

Hartman DS, Davis CJ Jr, Goldman SM, Friedman AC, Fritzsche P. Renal lymphoma: radiologic-pathologic correlation of 21 cases. *Radiol* 1982; **144**: 759–766.

Hayden CK Jr, Swischuk LE. Renal cystic disease. *Semin Ultrasound CT MR* 1991; **12**: 361–373.

Hernanz-Schulman M. Hyperechoic renal medullary pyramids in infants and children. *Radiol* 1991; **181**: 9–11.

Hoffer FA, Hanabergh AM, Teele RL. The interrenicular junction: a mimic of renal scarring on normal pediatric sonograms. *AJR* 1985; **145**: 1075–1078.

Jayagopal S, Cohen HL, Bhagat J, Eaton DH. Hyperechoic renal cortical masses: an unusual sonographic presentation of acute lymphoblastic leukemia in a child. *J Clin Ultrasound* 1991; **19**: 425–429.

Jayagopal S, Cohen HL, Brill PW, Winchester P, Eaton D. Calcified neonatal renal vein thrombosis demonstration by CT and US. *Pediatr Radiol* 1990; **20**: 160–162.

Jequier S, Rousseau O. Sonographic measurements of the normal bladder wall in children. *AJR* 1987; **149**: 563–566.

Kaude JV, Lacy GD. Ultrasonography in renal lymphoma. *J Clin Ultrasound* 1978; **6**: 321–323.

Kessler RM, Quevedo H, Lankau CA, et al. Obstructive vs. non-obstructive dilatation of the renal collecting system in children: distinction with duplex sonography. *AJR* 1993; **160**: 353–357.

Kier R, Taylor KJW, Feyock AL, Ramos IM. Renal masses: characterization with Doppler US. *Radiol* 1990; **176**: 703–707.

Kirpekar M, Abiri MM, Hilfer C, Enerson R. Ultrasound in the diagnosis of systemic candidiasis (renal and cranial) in very low birth weight premature infants. *Pediatr Radiol* 1986; **16**: 17–20.

Laplante S, Patriquin HB, Robitaille P, Filiatrault D, Grignon A, Decarie J-C. Renal vein thrombosis in children: evidence of early flow recovery with Doppler US. *Radiology* 1993; **189**: 37–42.

Lebowitz RL. The detection of vesicoureteral reflux in the child. *Invest Radiol* 1986; **21**: 519–531.

Marshall JL, Johnson ND, De Campo MP. Vesicoureteric reflux in children: prediction with color Doppler imaging. *Radiology* 1990; **175**: 355–358.

McHugh K, Stringer DA, Hebert D, Babiak CA. Simple renal cysts in children: diagnosis and follow-up with US. *Radiology* 1991; **178**: 383–385.

Meyer JS, Lebowitz RL. Primary megaureter in infants and children: a review. *Urol Radiol* 1992; **14**: 296–305.

Middleton WD, Dodds WJ, Lawson TL, Foley WD. Renal calculi: sensitivity for detection with US. *Radiology* 1988; **167**: 239–244.

Narla LD, Slovis TL, Watts FB, Nigro M. The renal lesions of tuberosclerosis (cysts and angiomyolipoma) – screening with sonography and computerized tomography. *Pediatr Radiol* 1988; **18**: 205–209.

Parvey HR, Eisenberg RL. Image-directed Doppler sonography of the intrarenal arteries in acute renal vein thrombosis. *J Clin Ultrasound* 1990; **18**: 512–516.

Patriquin H. Doppler examination of the kidney in infants and children. *Urol Radiol* 1991; **12**: 220–227.

Patriquin HB, O'Regan S. Medullary sponge kidney in childhood. *AJR* 1985; **145**: 315–319.

Platt JF, Rubin JM, Ellis JH. Acute renal obstruction: evaluation with intrarenal duplex Doppler and conventional US. *Radiol* 1993; **186**: 685–688.

Pollack HM, Wein AJ. Imaging of renal trauma. *Radiol* 1989; **172**: 297–308.

Pozniak MA, Kelcz F, Dodd GD III. Renal transplant ultrasound: imaging and Doppler. *Semin Ultrasound CT MR* 1991; **12**: 319–334.

Premkumar A, Berdon WE, Levy J, Amodio J, Abramson SJ, Newhouse JH. The emergence of hepatic fibrosis and portal hypertension in infants and children with autosomal recessive polycystic kidney disease. Initial and follow-up sonographic and radiographic findings. *Pediatr Radiol* 1988; **18**: 123–129.

Rosenbaum DM, Karngold E, Teele RL. Sonographic assessment of renal length in normal children *AJR* 1984; 142: 467–469.

Sanders RC, Hartman DS. The sonographic distinction between neonatal multicystic kidney and hydronephrosis. *Radiol* 1984; **151**: 621–625.

Sanders RC, Nussbaum AR, Solez K. Renal dysplasia: sonographic findings. *Radiol* 1988; **167**: 623–626.

Schaffer RM, Shih YH, Becker JA. Sonographic identification of collecting system duplications. *J Clin Ultrasound* 1983; **11**: 309–312.

Schlesinger AE, Hernandez RJ, Zerin JM, Marks TI, Kelsch RC. Interobserver and intraobserver variations in sonographic renal length measurements in children. *AJR* 1991; **156**: 1029–1032.

Schneider K, Helmig FJ, Eife R, et al. Pyonephrosis in childhood – is ultrasound sufficient for diagnosis? *Pediatr Radiol* 1989; **19**: 302–307.

Shultz PK, Strife JL, Strife CF, McDaniel JD. Hyperechoic renal medullary pyramids in infants and children. *Radiol* 1991; **181**: 163–167.

Siegel MJ Ed. *Pediatric Sonography*. 2nd ed. New York: Raven Press; 1995.

Stuck KJ, Silver TM, Jaffe MH, Bowerman RA. Sonographic demonstration of renal fungus balls. *Radiol* 1981; **142**: 473–474.

Surratt JT, Siegel MJ, Middleton WD. Sonography of complications in pediatric renal allografts. *Radiographics* 1990; **10**: 687–699.

Wood BP. Renal cystic disease in infants and children. *Urol Radial* 1992; 14: 284–293.

12

THE
FEMALE PELVIS

PREPARATION

Fluids should be given to achieve an adequately distended urinary bladder.

TRANSDUCER

Curvilinear transducer, the frequency dependent on patient build.

A high frequency linear transducer may aid visualisation of the uterus and ovaries in the neonate.

TECHNIQUE

Patient supine. The transducer is placed in the midline immediately superior to the symphysis pubis. The uterus is imaged in sequential longitudinal and transverse sections. The ovaries are more easily identified in transverse section, i.e. in the plane at 90 degrees to the long axis of the uterus. Cranial and caudal angulation will allow visualisation of each sovary in transverse section. The longitudinal section is best achieved by the contralateral approach using the urinary bladder as an acoustic window. The right ovary is imaged from the left side of the pelvis and vice versa for the left ovary.

NB. Transvaginal imaging of the female pelvis is not normally performed in children.

UTERUS

Normal ultrasound appearances

Prepubertal

- Smooth in outline, piriform in shape.

- Homogeneous, hypoechoic echotexture, interrupted centrally by the endometrium, a thin echogenic line.

Birth

Uterus appears prominent due to the influence of maternal hormones (Fig. 12.1).

Neonatal period

- The fundus becomes smaller than the cervix. The fundus accounts for one third of the length and the cervix the remaining two thirds. Remains unchanged in appearance until approximately 7 years.

- No obvious endometrial echo (Fig. 12.2).

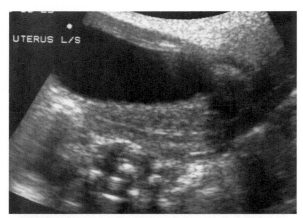

Figure 12.1 — The normal prominent neonatal uterus, with a thin echogenic line centrally representing the endometrial cavity.

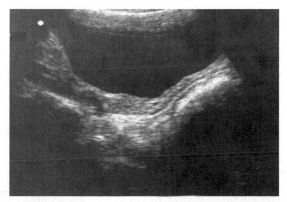

Figure 12.2 — The normal uterus in a 4-year-old demonstrating a small, tubular structure, with no distinction between the cervix and fundus.

Over 7 years

- Gradual increase in uterine size until puberty when it assumes a more 'adult' configuration.

- The fundus is large in comparison to the cervix (Fig. 12.3).

Postpubertal

- Lies in the midline, usually in an anteverted position (Fig. 12.4a) but can also be retroverted (Fig. 12.4b) or angled in its mid portion anteflexed or retroflexed (Fig. 12.4c).

- Smooth in outline, piriform in shape.

- Homogeneous hypoechoic echotexture.

- The appearance of the endometrium changes with the menstrual cycle.

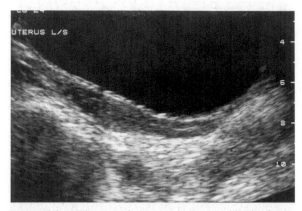

Figure 12.3 — The normal uterus in a 10-year-old. The fundus and cervix can now be distinguished. The endometrial cavity is seen as an echogenic line centrally continuous with the vaginal cavity.

Menstrual phase

- Degenerating: irregular relatively hypoechoic texture, with thickness dependent on the day of menstruation.

- Blood in the uterine cavity may be seen as an anechoic area.

Early proliferative phase

Weak, thin echogenic linear echo (Fig. 12.5a).

Late proliferative phase

- Gradually increases in thickness during the proliferative phase.

- Immediately after ovulation the 'ring sign' is present; the endometrium appears hypoechoic centrally surrounded by an echogenic rim (Fig. 12.5b).

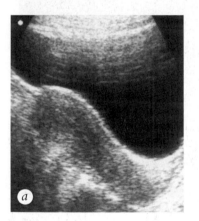
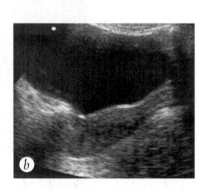
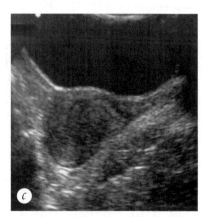

Figure 12.4 — Pubertal uterus: examples of normal uterine positions: (a) anteverted (b) retroverted (c) retroflexed.

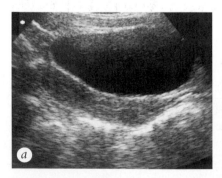
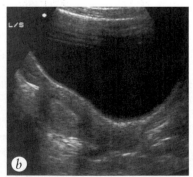
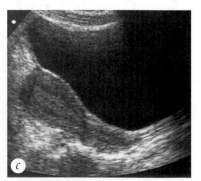

Figure 12.5 — (a) The adult configuration of the uterus which is pear-shaped due to the altered ratio of fundus to cervix. The thin endometrial echo indicates the early proliferative phase. (b) Late proliferative phase: the 'ring-sign' is seen immediately after ovulation; the endometrium appears hypoechoic centrally and is surrounded by an echogenic rim. (c) The secretory phase: the endometrium appears thickened and echogenic.

Secretory phase

The endometrium gradually increases in echogenicity and thickness until menstruation occurs (Fig. 12.5c).

Uterine size

Best assessed by calculating the volume using the formula for the volume of an ellipsoid: length × anteroposterior diameter × transverse diameter × 0.5 (Table 12.1).

Table 12.1 Uterine volume in relation to age

Age	Volume	
0–1 month	3.4	(1.2)
3 months	0.9	(0.2)
1 year	1.0	(0.2)
3 years	1.0	(0.3)
5 years	1.0	(0.3)
7 years	0.9	(0.3)
9 years	1.3	(0.4)
11 years	1.9	(0.9)
13 years	11.0	(10.5)
15 years	21.2	(13.5)

Values are the mean (SD) in millilitres.

(Adapted from: *Ultrasound Evaluation of Uterine and Ovarian Size from Birth to Puberty.* H.P. Haber, E.I. Mayer.)

Normal ultrasound appearances of the vagina

- Extends from the cervix to the introitus (Fig. 12.6a).

- Hypoechoic tubular structure in longitudinal section with an echogenic linear echo centrally, representing the opposing inner walls.

- In transverse section, oval in shape, increasing in diameter towards the cervix.

PITFALL

Fluid is sometimes seen in the vagina post micturition or if the bladder is over-distended: urine refluxes into the vagina. This will resolve if the patient is scanned after standing erect (Fig. 12.6b).

Congenital anomalies

Uterine agenesis

Absence of the uterus is rare but is seen in testicular feminisation (46XY karyotype).

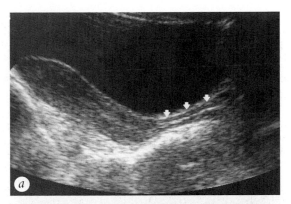

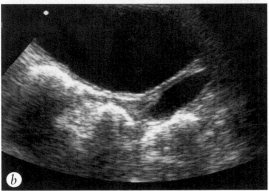

Figure 12.6 — (a) The normal vagina: Hypoechoic tubular structure continuous with the cervix and uterus with an echogenic linear echo centrally representing the opposing inner walls. (b) Reflux of urine into the vagina causing mild dilatation of its cavity.

Outwardly these children have female genitalia but the vagina ends blindly as the cervix and uterus are absent. The gonads are testes, located in the pelvis or inguinal canal.

Not usually diagnosed until puberty when the child presents with primary amenorrhoea.

Uterine hypoplasia

Small uterus (Fig. 12.7).

Diagnosis usually made at puberty.

CAUSES

Lack of oestrogen produced due to pituitary/hypothalamic or ovarian failure.

Turner's syndrome, mosaic Turner's syndrome.

Diethylstilbestrol exposure in utero.

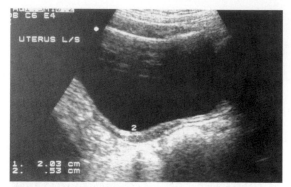

Figure 12.7 — Small hypoplastic uterus measuring 2.0 × 0.5 cm in an 11-year-old girl with Turner's syndrome.

Uterine duplication

Various anomalies occur due to incomplete fusion of mullerian ducts in prenatal life.

Examples include:

Uterus didelphys – two vaginas, two cervices, two uterine bodies.

Uterus bicornis bicollis – one vagina, two cervices, two uterine bodies.

Uterus bicornis unicollis (bicornuate uterus) – one vagina, one cervix, two uterine horns (Fig. 12.8).

Uterus unicornis unicollis – unilateral failure of development.

Uterus septus – single uterus divided by a septum.

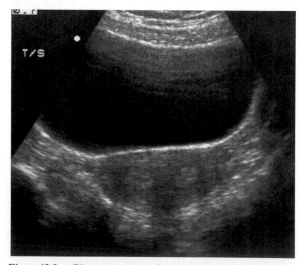

Figure 12.8 — Bicornuate uterus. A transverse section through the fundus of the uterus demonstrating two separate endometrial echoes.

Congenital absence of the vagina

Rare.

Seen in association with absence or anomalies of the uterus, e.g. Mayer-Rokitansky-Küster-Hauser syndrome – hypoplastic or absent vagina with a variety of uterine anomalies, associated with renal and skeletal abnormalities.

Congenital vaginal obstruction

May result from:

Vaginal atresia, when it is usually associated with other anomalies, e.g. bicornuate uterus, renal anomalies, imperforate anus.

Imperforate hymen, an isolated finding.

TYPES OF OBSTRUCTION

Hydrocolpos – only the vagina is involved.

Hydrometrocolpos – both the uterus and vagina are dilated.

Haematometrocolpos – both the uterus and vagina are dilated and the discharge is bloody.

CLINICAL PRESENTATION

Symptoms cause presentation in the newborn and more commonly at puberty.

In the neonatal period

A palpable abdominal mass which is a combination of bladder and fluid-filled vagina.

A bulging mass at the introitus may be present.

At puberty

Amenorrhoea.

Abdominal pain, often cyclical in nature as menstruation takes place into the obstructed vagina

Ultimately, pain and pelvic mass.

PITFALL

In children with a double uterus and vagina, one horn and vagina may be patent so the child menstruates normally but still presents with pain.

Ultrasound findings are similar except that a 'normal' uterine horn may be seen.

MR is needed to identify the anatomy properly.

ULTRASOUND APPEARANCES

Neonate

- Tubular in shape (Fig. 12.9).

- Mainly cystic mass between the bladder and rectum.

- May contain low-level echoes.

- Fluid–debris level, often seen.

Puberty

- Large pelvic mass (Fig. 12.10a, b).

- Hypoechoic with low-level echoes representing blood.

- Fluid–debris level may be seen.

- May extend to involve Fallopian tubes.

- If very large, may obstruct the ureters, resulting in hydronephrosis.

Tumour: rhabdomyosarcoma

Most common malignant tumour of the vagina and uterus.

Usually arises from the anterior wall of the vagina, in females under 4 years old.

May involve bladder and other pelvic structures.

Uterus less commonly the site and usually occurs in older, pubertal girls.

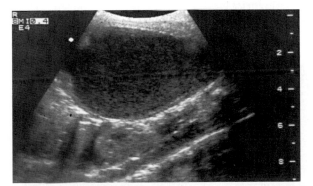

Figure 12.9 — A longitudinal section of the uterus and vagina in a one-day-old neonate demonstrating a cystic mass containing low-level echoes consistent with neonatal hydrometrocolpos.

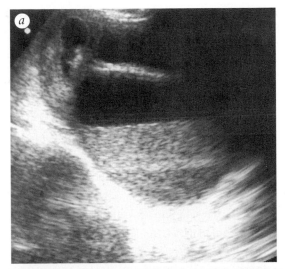

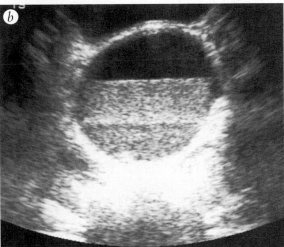

Figure 12.10 — Haematometrocolpos. (a) Longitudinal section of the uterus and vagina in a 13-year-old girl. The vagina is dilated, appearing mainly cystic with fluid/debris levels. The uterus is seen superiorly with a small amount of fluid in its cavity. (b) Transverse section through the vagina of the same patient.

CLINICAL PRESENTATION

Vaginal origin

Vaginal mass.

Discharge/bleeding, often thought to be haematuria.

May cause hydronephrosis due to ureteral obstruction.

Difficulty in micturition.

Anuria.

If large, may prolapse through the vagina.

Uterine origin
Abdominal mass.

ULTRASOUND APPEARANCES (Fig. 12.11)

- Heterogeneous, hyperechoic mass arising from uterus/vagina.

- Hypoechoic areas if there is necrosis.

- Associated findings
  - ascites
  - lymphadenopathy
  - liver metastases
  - local extension into adjacent structures.

CT/MR required to determine full extent of the disease.

Other uterine and vaginal neoplasms are rare in children, and need tissue diagnosis by biopsy. They include lymphoma, endometrial and cervical carcinoma.

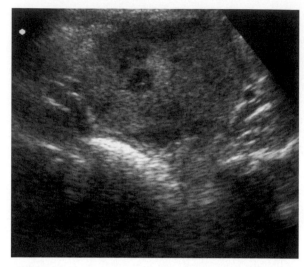

Figure 12.11 — Rhabdomyosarcoma. Transverse section through the pelvis demonstrating a large well-circumscribed predominantly hyperechoic mass with hypoechoic areas suggestive of necrosis.

OVARIES

Normal ultrasound appearances

Pre-pubertal

- The ovaries are positioned in the superior margin of the broad ligament.

- Oval in shape.

Neonates/young infants (Fig. 12.12a)
Small follicles (less than 7 mm in diameter, well-defined anechoic structures) scattered through the ovarian stroma, due to the influence of maternal hormones.

Under 5 years (Fig. 12.12b)
Homogeneous echotexture.

Over 5 years (Fig. 12.12c)
Small follicles less than 7 mm in diameter.

Number of follicles increases with age.

Follicles are scattered throughout the ovarian stroma.

A gradual increase in ovarian size is seen as puberty approaches.

Puberty

- The ovaries are positioned deeper in the pelvis, superiorly and laterally to the uterus with the bladder distended. The uterine artery can be used as a landmark.

- Appearances vary with the menstrual cycle.

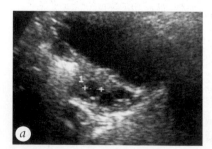
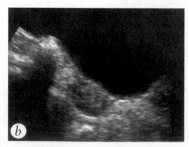
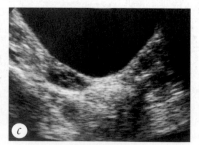

Figure 12.12 — (a) Small 6 mm diameter follicles are scattered throughout the ovarian stroma in a neonate. (b) The normal homogeneous echotexture of the ovary in a 4-year-old. (c) The normal ovary in a 10-year-old with small follicles scattered throughout the ovarian stroma.

Follicular phase (day 1–13 assuming a 28-day cycle)
Follicles gradually increase in size due to the influence of FSH (follicle stimulating hormone); by day 8–9, a dominant follicle is evident which continues to develop (up to 3 cm in diameter) until ovulation occurs (Fig. 12.13a).

Ovulation
Follicular size reduces and may have irregular walls (crenation)

+/– Free fluid in the Pouch of Douglas.

Post ovulation (Fig. 12.13b)
Small unstimulated follicles throughout the ovarian stroma.

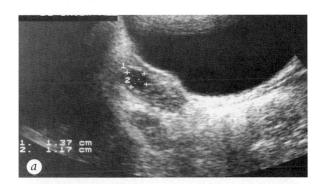

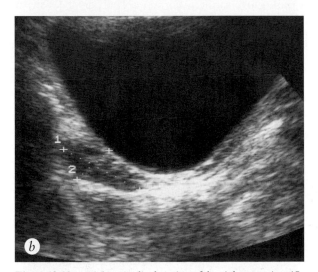

Figure 12.13 — (a) Longitudinal section of the right ovary in a 15-year-old (day 11 of the menstrual cycle) with a single dominant follicle measuring 1.4 × 1.2 cm. (b) Secretory phase ovary: following ovulation, multiple small unstimulated follicles are evident throughout the ovarian stroma.

Ovarian size

Best assessed by calculating the volume, using the formula for an ellipsoid, length × anteroposterior diameter × transverse diameter × 0.5 (Table 12.2).

Table 12.2 Ovarian volume in relation to age

Age	Volume	
0–1 month	0.5	(0.4)
3 months	0.4	(0.1)
1 year	0.5	(0.2)
3 years	0.7	(0.4)
5 years	0.7	(0.5)
7 years	0.8	(0.6)
9 years	0.6	(0.4)
11 years	1.3	(1.0)
13 years	3.7	(2.1)
15 years	6.7	(4.8)

Values are the mean (SD) in millilitres.
(Adapted from: *Ultrasound Evaluation of Uterine and Ovarian Size from Birth to Puberty.* H.P. Haber, E.I. Mayer.)

Congenital anomalies

Absence

Always check the inguinal canals for the possibility of herniation.

Dysplasia

Seen in Turner's syndrome and mosaic Turner's (Fig. 12.14).

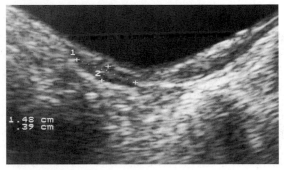

Figure 12.14 — Small 'streak-like' ovary seen in an 11-year-old with Turner's syndrome.

Turner's: ovaries appear streak-like. Secondary sexual characteristics do not develop at puberty. The uterus remains pre-pubertal.

Mosaic Turner's: ovaries appear small or almost normal in size. Secondary sexual characteristics develop at puberty including menstruation.

Polycystic ovaries (Stein-Leventhal syndrome)

The syndrome is associated with:

Amenorrhoea

Infertility

Hirsutism

Obesity.

CLINICAL PRESENTATION

The above conditions.

ULTRASOUND APPEARANCES (Fig. 12.15)

- Bilaterally enlarged ovaries (but can be normal in size).
- 10 or more cysts less than 8 mm in diameter, with increased ovarian stroma.
- Cysts are arranged around the periphery of the ovary: 'string of pearls' appearance.
- Hypoechoic/isoechoic appearance of the ovaries when compared to the uterus.

LIMITATIONS

Adolescent ovaries often appear to contain multiple follicles and therefore the diagnosis can only be made in conjunction with the appropriate endocrine tests.

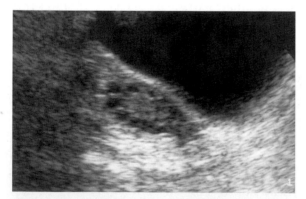

Figure 12.15 — Multiple follicles located around the periphery of the left ovary – the 'string of pearls' appearance typical of polycystic ovary disease.

Ovarian cysts (Fig. 12.16)

Follicular cysts

A result of continued hormonal stimulation of a follicle that does not rupture at ovulation.

CLINICAL PRESENTATION

Asymptomatic, often an incidental finding.

If large, may present as a palpable mass.

Pain due to

- haemorrhage
- torsion
- rupture.

ULTRASOUND APPEARANCES

- Well-defined.
- Anechoic, with acoustic enhancement.
- May contain septae.
- Size variable, usually more than 3 cm.
- Free fluid in the Pouch of Douglas following resolution.

TREATMENT

Conservative as the majority resolve spontaneously. A re-scan at a different phase in the menstrual cycle should be performed to check the cyst has resolved.

Complications of a follicular cyst include torsion and haemorrhage.

Haemorrhagic cysts

Haemorrhagic cysts are a complication of a follicular cyst.

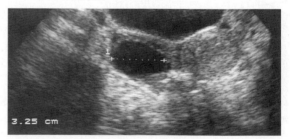

Figure 12.16 — Transverse section of the right ovary containing a 3 cm diameter simple cyst – a result of continued hormonal stimulation of a follicle that has not ruptured at ovulation.

CLINICAL PRESENTATION
Acute lower abdominal/pelvic pain.

ULTRASOUND APPEARANCES (Fig. 12.17a–c)

- Appearance variable, depending on the state of blood within the cyst. Fresh blood is anechoic. As clot forms, it appears more hyperechoic/echogenic.

- Complex mass demonstrating acoustic enhancement.

- Echotexture – heterogeneous/homogeneous.

- Echogenicity – hypo/hyperechoic.

- Fluid/fluid level, fluid/debris level.

- +/– thick wall.

- +/– septae.

- +/– free fluid in the Pouch of Douglas.

LIMITATIONS
It is often hard to distinguish from other ovarian pathologies, e.g. ovarian torsion, abscess, teratoma, cyst –adenoma and tumour. If acute surgical conditions, e.g. torsion, appendicitis, can be excluded serial ultrasound examinations should be performed. The appearance of a haemorrhagic cyst changes with time.

Torsion of an ovarian cyst

CLINICAL PRESENTATION
As for haemorrhagic cyst.

ULTRASOUND APPEARANCES
Similar to a haemorrhagic cyst and it may be impossible to differentiate the two with ultrasound. However, the appearance of a torted cyst does not usually change over a few days whereas the appearance of a haemorrhagic cyst changes as clot forms and resolution occurs.

Neonatal cysts

Usually follicular in origin and due to stimulation by maternal hormones.

CLINICAL PRESENTATION

- Antenatal diagnosis.

- Abdominal mass.

ULTRASOUND APPEARANCES (Fig. 12.18)

- Large simple cyst.

- Well-defined.

- Thin-walled.

- Acoustic enhancement.

- +/– hydronephrosis due to pressure on the ureters.

- May contain internal echoes, +/– fluid/debris levels.

LIMITATIONS
Due to the small size of the infant pelvis, neonatal ovarian cysts lie within the abdominal cavity and their pelvic origin is not always obvious.

COMPLICATIONS
Haemorrhage

Torsion.

TREATMENT
Ultrasound follow-up is advised and treatment depends on the size. Less than 5 cm usually resolve spontaneously. More than 5 cm may require aspiration.

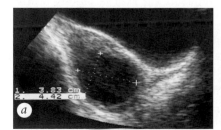
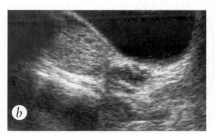
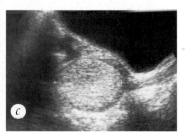

Figure 12.17 — Haemorrhagic cyst. (a) A cystic mass within the left adnexa containing fine internal echoes. (b) A well-defined homogeneous hyperechoic mass adjacent to the left ovary. (c) A well-defined echogenic mass. All examples demonstrate a degree of post-cystic enhancement.

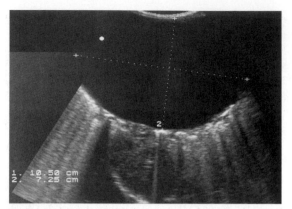

Figure 12.18 — A large thin-walled cystic mass arising from the pelvis in a 1-day-old neonate.

Ovarian torsion

The adnexae in children are very mobile. Torsion results from the partial or complete rotation of the ovary on its pedicle.

More common in prepubertal girls and when there is an underlying abnormality, e.g. cyst, tumour.

CLINICAL PRESENTATION

Acute lower abdominal or pelvic pain.

Palpable mass.

Nausea, vomiting.

Leukocytosis.

Anorexia.

A previous history of episodes of similar pain.

It is often difficult to distinguish clinically from other acute conditions, e.g. appendicitis.

ULTRASOUND APPEARANCES (Fig. 12.19)
- Complex mass.
- Enlargement of the ovary.
- Multiple enlarged follicles (8–12 mm in diameter) peripherally located. (Circulatory impairment results in congestion of the ovary and transudation of fluid into follicles.)
- +/– free fluid in the Pouch of Douglas.
- +/– underlying abnormality, e.g. cyst/tumour.
- No obvious blood flow on colour flow imaging.

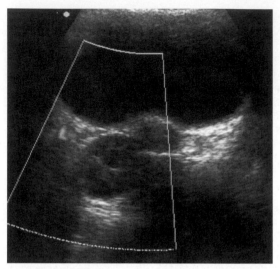

Figure 12.19 — Ovarian torsion. The right ovary appears enlarged with multiple enlarged follicles and no obvious colour flow.

Tumours

Uncommon in childhood.

Benign tumours are seen in all ages, but are more common in pre-pubertal girls.

Malignant tumours are more commonly seen after puberty.

Benign

CLINICAL PRESENTATION

Abdominal pain.

Palpable mass.

Abdominal distension.

Constipation.

Genito-urinary symptoms, e.g. hydronephrosis, urinary frequency.

Acute signs if torsion or rupture occurs.

Cystadenoma

Two types: mucinous and serous (more common).

Rare in children, usually more than 20 years, but sometimes seen in postpubertal females.

Size variable: 4–20 cm.

May undergo malignant change.

ULTRASOUND APPEARANCES (Fig. 12.20)

- Well-defined.

- Mainly cystic.

- Often large.

- Serous type may
  - contain septae
  - be bilateral
  - have internal echoes.

- Mucinous type may
  - be unilateral
  - have multiple septae.

They can sometimes be difficult to distinguish from a simple cyst on ultrasound.

Germ cell tumours

Include dermoids, a benign tumour, and teratomas, which in the pelvis are usually benign but can be malignant.

Rare under 2 years.

Occasionally bilateral.

Vary in size: 5–25 cm.

ULTRASOUND APPEARANCES (Fig. 12.21a–c)

- Extremely variable, depends on composition, e.g. hair, fat, calcification, cartilage appear echogenic, serous fluid/sebum appears hypoechoic.

- May appear as a complex mass with hypoechoic echogenic components or a mainly cystic mass. Both usually well-defined.

- 'Iceberg' – echogenic material may cause acoustic shadowing, resulting in the inability to visualise the whole of the lesion.

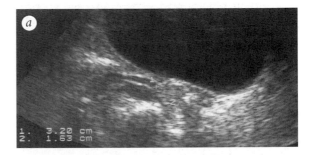
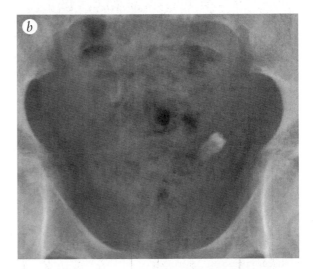
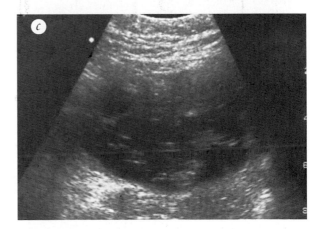

Figure 12.21 — Ovarian dermoid. (a) A hyperechoic mass with a central echogenic area casting an acoustic shadow suggesting an area of calcification within it. (b) An abdominal X-ray of the same patient revealed this to be a 'tooth'. (c) A cystic mass with some echogenic contents which, following investigation, was confirmed as a benign teratoma.

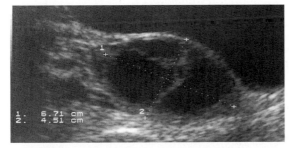

Figure 12.20 — Cystadenoma. A well-defined cystic mass in the right adnexa containing multiple septae.

- Mainly echogenic lesions – may be difficult to distinguish from neighbouring bowel. Look for associated sign, e.g. mass effect indentation of the urinary bladder.

- Fluid/fluid levels, fluid/fat levels.

- A large mass may cause pressure on the ureters resulting in hydronephrosis.

- If malignant, tends to be a more solid lesion; confirmed if there are liver metastases, malignant ascites or lymphadenopathy.

NB. Ascites may also occur with benign lesions if they rupture into the peritoneum.

Malignant

Rare, usually occur after puberty.

Most common in paediatric age group is dysgerminoma.

CLINICAL PRESENTATION

Abdominal pain.

Palpable mass.

Abdominal distension.

Nausea, vomiting, anorexia.

ULTRASOUND APPEARANCES (Fig. 12.22)

- Irregular outline.

- Usually predominantly solid, or mixed solid and cystic.

- Contain septae.

- Free fluid in the Pouch of Douglas.

- If advanced
  - local extension
  - ascites
  - liver metastases
  - lymphadenopathy.

Secondary neoplasms

Lymphoma, leukaemia and neuroblastomas may all infiltrate the ovaries causing diffuse enlargement.

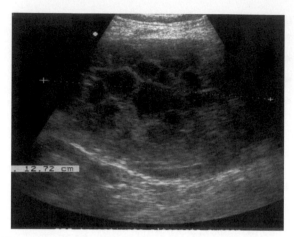

Figure 12.22 — Malignant ovarian mass. A large, well-defined mixed solid and cystic lesion.

Other malignant tumours of the pelvis, e.g. rhabdomyosarcomas, may involve the ovaries due to local extension.

Precocious puberty

Premature development of secondary sexual characteristics.

- Breast development, gonadal enlargement, the presence of pubic/axillary hair before 8 years

- Menstruation before 9 years.

True precocious puberty

All the secondary sexual characteristics are present.

CAUSES

Early hormonal stimulation.

Lesions of the central nervous system, e.g. pituitary, hypothalamus.

Pseudo precocious puberty

Some of the secondary sexual characteristics are present, but not ovulation.

CAUSE

A hormonally active lesion arising from the adrenal or ovary.

THE ROLE OF ULTRASOUND

Assess the volume and endometrial status of the uterus.

Assess ovarian volume and follicular size.

Exclude or confirm the presence of an adrenal or ovarian mass.

ULTRASOUND APPEARANCES

True precocious puberty (Fig. 12.23 a, b)
- Adult/pubertal appearances of the uterus and ovaries.

Pseudo precocious puberty
- Variable.

- Prepubertal/developing/pubertal uterus.

- Asymmetrical or symmetrical enlargement of the ovaries.

- Ovarian cysts.

- Ovarian or adrenal mass.

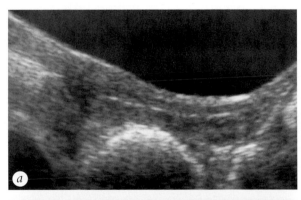

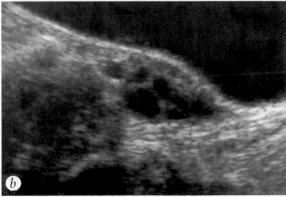

Figure 12.23 — Precocious puberty. Pubertal appearances (a & b) of the uterus and ovaries in an 8-year-old girl.

Following effective treatment ultrasound can be performed to ensure the uterus and ovaries are prepubertal in configuration.

Pregnancy

A possible cause of a pelvic mass in adolescent girls.

CLINICAL PRESENTATION

Pelvic mass.

Abdominal/pelvic pain.

Vomiting/nausea.

Amenorrhoea.

Following a positive pregnancy test, ultrasound should be performed to

Confirm the diagnosis.

Establish that the pregnancy is intrauterine.

Determine maturity.

Confirm viability.

ULTRASOUND APPEARANCES (Fig. 12.24)

Variable, depending on maturity.

- < 6 weeks: a gestational sac is demonstrated within the uterus.

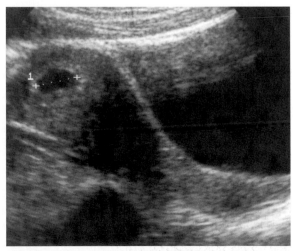

Figure 12.24 — Pregnancy. A longitudinal section of the uterus demonstrating a gestational sac at approximately 5 weeks. The fetal pole is not yet visible.

- > 6 weeks: the embryo and fetal heart movement are visible within the gestational sac. A crown–rump length is the most accurate method of dating between 6–12 weeks.

- > 12 weeks: A bi-parietal diameter should be performed to determine maturity.

Referral to a dedicated obstetric centre is necessary following a positive diagnosis.

Ectopic pregnancy

A potentially fatal complication of pregnancy. The pregnancy is located outside the uterine cavity.

CLINICAL PRESENTATION

Abdominal/pelvic pain.

A history of missed or irregular periods.

Palpable mass.

Positive pregnancy test.

Shock (if rupture has occurred).

ULTRASOUND APPEARANCES

- No evidence of an intrauterine pregnancy.

- A solid/complex adnexal mass.

- A decidual reaction in the uterus, the endometrium appears echogenic.

- Free fluid in the Pouch of Douglas.

The ultrasound examination may be normal, if it is an early pregnancy and rupture has not occurred.

Laparoscopy may confirm or exclude an ectopic pregnancy when the ultrasound findings are equivocal.

Pelvic inflammatory disease

Infection of the pelvis, which in adolescents is more common in those who are sexually active. The most common causes are gonorrhoea and chlamydia. Infection spreads along the mucous membranes from the vulva to the adnexa. The Fallopian tube is the most common site of localisation.

CLINICAL PRESENTATION

Febrile.

Vaginal discharge +/– purulent.

Pelvic pain.

Cervical motion tenderness.

+/– palpable mass.

ULTRASOUND APPEARANCES (Fig. 12.25)

May be normal but possible findings include:

Acute salpingitis

Inflammation of the Fallopian tube. Free fluid is seen in the Pouch of Douglas.

Pyosalpinx

The Fallopian tube is blocked and pus accumulates. A hypoechoic tubular mass with internal echoes.

Hydrosalpinx

Pus from a pyosalpinx is reabsorbed, resulting in a sterile watery fluid. An anechoic tubular collection may be difficult to differentiate from an ovarian cyst.

Tubo ovarian abscess

A collection of pus which envelops both the Fallopian tube and ovary. Ultrasound appearances are variable.

- Thick irregular walls.

- Echogenic.

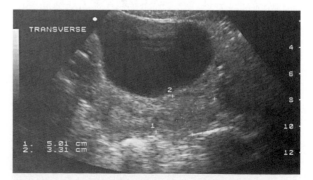

Figure 12.25 — Pelvic inflammatory disease. A complex mass in the left adnexa involving the left ovary and Fallopian tube in a 15-year-old.

- Anechoic areas if liquefaction or necrosis occurs.
- Fluid/debris levels.
- Septae.
- Free fluid in the Pouch of Douglas.

Pelvic abscess

An abscess forms behind the uterus or in the region of the ovary. An ill-defined complex mass. May be confused with appendicitis.

Treatment

Antibiotics but occasionally surgical drainage is required.

Other pelvic masses

Presacral

Sometimes confused with uterine or ovarian masses.

Sacrococcygeal teratoma

A germ cell tumour which occurs in the presacral region. Early diagnosis and treatment is necessary as it has a malignant tendency. There are 4 types, classified as follows:

Type I – Mainly external with a small presacral component.

Type II – External with a significant intrapelvic component.

Type III – Mainly internal (pelvic and abdominal) with a small external component.

Type IV – Entirely presacral.

CLINICAL PRESENTATION

A large mass with or without an external component.

Types I–III usually present at birth.

Type IV may present later as there is no external evidence of the mass. It may be small initially but becomes large when there is malignant change.

ULTRASOUND APPEARANCES (Fig. 12.26a, b)
- Variable.
- Echogenic/anechoic/complex mass.

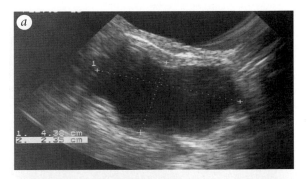

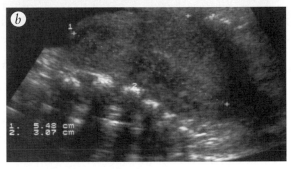

Figure 12.26 — (a) Benign sacrococcygeal teratoma in an 11-day-old girl. A longitudinal section through the pelvis demonstrates a predominantly cystic mass posterior to the bladder. (b) A large malignant sacrococcygeal teratoma with a large predominantly solid internal component anterior to the sacrum displacing the bladder superiorly.

- Hydronephrosis, due to compression or involvement of the ureters or bladder.

OTHER IMAGING

MRI is the imaging modality of choice to determine the total extent of the mass.

A plain radiograph may demonstrate calcification or fat.

Presacral neuroblastoma (Fig. 12.27)
Arises in the neuronal tissue extra-adrenally.

Occurs in young infants and young children.

CLINICAL PRESENTATION
Pain.

Palpable mass.

Constipation.

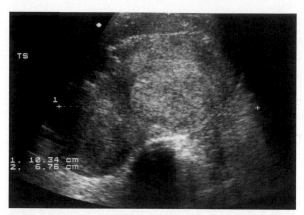

Figure 12.27 — Neuroblastoma. A large well-defined complex mass arising from the pelvis.

Urinary frequency or obstruction.

Neurological signs if spinal infiltration with cord involvement takes place.

ULTRASOUND APPEARANCES

- Mainly solid or complex mass.

Lymphoma

If the pelvis is involved, pelvic nodes appear as homogeneous, hypoechoic well-defined lesions. They may cause indentation of the bladder. The liver, spleen and kidneys should also be assessed for evidence of infiltration.

Pelvic abscess

In children, ruptured appendix or a postoperative collection are the common causes. See appendicitis for further details.

Anterior sacral meningocele

Rare anomaly.

Presacral cystic mass.

May be confused on ultrasound with ovarian cysts.

Sacral dysraphism on pelvic X-ray.

CLINICAL PRESENTATION

Neurological symptoms if there is spinal cord tethering.

Palpable mass.

If infected, ascending meningitis.

ULTRASOUND APPEARANCES

- Presacral cystic mass.

- May have associated neuropathic anomalies of the kidneys and bladder – hydronephrosis and reflux nephropathy.

Further reading

Babcock DS, Hann BK. The pediatric pelvis. *Clin Diagn Ultrasound* 1984; **15**: 27–46.

Bass IS, Haller JO, Friedman AP, Twersky J, Balsam D, Gotteman R. The sonographic appearance of the hemorrhagic ovarian cyst in adolescents. *J Ultrasound Med* 1984; **3**: 509–513.

Blask ARN, Sanders RC, Gearhart JP. Obstructed uterovaginal anomalies: demonstration with sonography. Part I: neonates and infants. *Radiology* 1991; **179**: 79–83.

Blask ARN, Sanders RC, Rock JA. Obstructed uterovaginal anomalies: demonstration with sonography. Part II: teen-agers. *Radiology* 1991; **179**: 84–88.

Brammer HM, Buck JL, Hayes WS, Sheth S, Tavassoli FA. Malignant germ cell tumors of the ovary: radiologic-pathologic correlation. *Radiographics* 1990; **10**: 715–724.

Breen JL, Bonamo JF, Maxson WS. Genital tract tumors in children. *Pediatr Clin North Am* 1981; **28**: 355–367.

Cohen HL, Bober SE, Bow SN. Imaging the pediatric pelvis: the normal and abnormal genital tract and simulators of its diseases. *Urol Radiol* 1992; **14**: 273–283.

Cohen HL, Eisenberg P, Mandel F, Haller JO. Ovarian cysts are common in premenarcheal girls: a sonographic study of 101 children 2–12 years old. *AJR* 1992; **159**: 89–91.

Cohen HL, Tice HM, Mandel FS. Ovarian volumes measured by US: bigger than we think. *Radiology* 1990; **177**: 189–192.

Haber HP, Mayer EI. Ultrasound evaluation of uterine and ovarian size from birth to puberty. *Pediatr Radiol* 1994; **24**: 11–13.

King LR, Siegel MJ, Solomon AL. The usefulness of ovarian volume and cysts in female isosexual precocious puberty. *J Ultrasound Med* 1993; **12**: 577–581.

Nussbaum AR, Sanders RC, Hartman DS, Dudgeon DL, Parmley TH. Neonatal ovarian cysts: sonographic-pathologic correlation. *Radiology* 1988; **168**: 817–821.

Rosenberg HK, Sherman NH, Tarry WF, Duckett JW, Synder HM, Mayer-Rokitansky-Kuster-Hauser syndrome: US aid to diagnosis. *Radiology* 1986; **161**: 815–819.

Siegel MJ. Pediatric gynecologic sonography. *Radiology* 1991; **179**: 593–600.

Surratt JT, Siegel MJ. Imaging of pediatric ovarian masses. *Radiographics* 1991; **11**: 533–548.

Thind C, Carty H and Pilling DW. The role of ultrasound in the management of ovarian masses in children. *Clin Rad* 1989; **40**: 180–182.

13

THE MALE GENITAL TRACT

Anatomy

The scrotum is a cutaneous outpouching of the abdomen consisting of loose skin and superficial fascia. It is the supporting structure for the testes. The scrotum internally is divided into 2 sacs each containing a single testis.

The testes are paired oval glands and develop high on the embryo's posterior abdominal wall, and usually enter the scrotum by 32 weeks' gestation. Full descent is not complete until just prior to birth. They lie in the scrotum with their long axis upright, tilted forward and slightly lateral. Each testis measures approximately 1.5 × 1.0 cm at birth and, as a result of a normal increase in testosterone levels during the first 3 months, increases in size to approximately 2.0 × 1.2 cm. The size of the testes then remains relatively constant until the age of 6 years when they again increase in size. After puberty, the testes measure 3–5 cm in length and 2–3 cm in width. The left testis is usually located slightly lower than the right.

The testis is covered by a layer of tissue called the tunica vaginalis, except for a small area posteriorly. This layer consists of 2 further layers which are separated by 1–2 ml of fluid. The inner layer of the tunica vaginalis is closely adherent to the fibrous capsule of the testis which is called the tunica albuginea. This layer invaginates into the testis to form a vertical septum of fibrous tissue called the mediastinum testis. Support for the arteries, veins and ducts is provided by the mediastinum testis as they enter and exit the testis.

The tunica albuginea divides each testis into a series of internal compartments called lobules. Each testis is composed of 200–300 lobules and each lobule contains 1–3 tightly coiled tubules called seminiferous tubules. These tubules are convoluted and as they course centrally they converge to form larger straight ducts called tubuli recti. These enter the mediastinum testis and form a network of channels called the rete testis. The rete testis in turn drains into the efferent ducts and then into the head of the epididymis.

The epididymis

The two epididymides are comma-shaped structures and lie along the posterolateral border of each testis. The epididymis consists of a tightly coiled tube, the ductus epididymis.

The larger, superior portion of the epididymis is known as the head. It continues into the epididymal body which tapers into the epididymal tail. The efferent ducts in the epididymal head empty into the ductus epididymis in the body of the epididymis. It continues into the epididymal tail as the ductus deferens (or seminal duct) and into the spermatic cord. The ductus deferens which is about 45 cm long ascends along the posterior border of the testis, penetrates the inguinal canal and enters the pelvic cavity where it loops down the posterior surface of the urinary bladder.

The spermatic cord

This structure supports the testicular artery, nerves, the pampiniform plexus of veins, lymphatics, the cremaster muscle along with the vas deferens. It passes through the inguinal canal, a slit-like passageway in the anterior abdominal wall just superior to the medial half of the inguinal ligament.

The testicular artery provides the main blood supply for the testis and is a branch of the abdominal aorta. It enters the spermatic cord at the deep inguinal ring. It courses along the posterior surface of the testis and forms capsular arteries just beneath the tunica albuginea. The deferential artery and cremasteric artery are also found in the spermatic cord and provide arterial supply to the epididymis, vas deferens and peritesticular tissues. The testicular deferential and cremasteric arteries converge at the mediastinum testis.

The pampiniform plexus, the draining veins of the testis, empty into the testicular veins. The right testicular vein empties into the inferior vena cava and the left drains into the left renal vein.

There are 3 main testicular appendages:

The appendix testis which is a remnant of the Müllerian duct and is attached to the upper pole of the testis.

The appendix epididymis which is a remnant of the mesonephron and is located on the head of the epididymis.

The vas aberrans which is a remnant of the mesonephron and is located between the body and tail of the epididymis.

CHOICE OF TRANSDUCER
10 MHz linear array.

PATIENT PREPARATION
None. In older children there should be great sensitivity with the boy who may be very embarrassed by the whole procedure.

Ultrasound appearances of normal testes

- Oval shaped structures of homogeneous low–medium echogenicity.

- Tunica albuginea seen as a thin echogenic line around each testis (Fig. 13.1).

- Mediastinum testis is seen within the testis, parallel to the epididymis as an echogenic line (Fig. 13.1).

- A small trace of fluid around each testis is a normal finding.

- The epididymal head is located posterolaterally to the superior pole of each testis, is triangular in shape and equal to or greater in echogenicity than that of the testis (Fig. 13.2).

- Epididymal body is equal to or less in echogenicity than that of the testis.

Birth to 3 months : the normal testis measures 1.5–2.0 cm in length and 1.0–1.2 cm in width.

Age 4–10 : normal testis measures 2 cm in length and 1.0–1.2 cm in width.

Age 11 upwards : normal testis measures 3–5 cm in length and 2–3 cm in width.

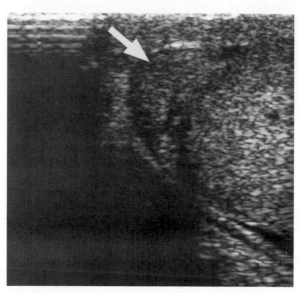

Figure 13.2 — Triangular-shaped epididymal head shown in longitudinal section.

TECHNIQUE

The patient is supine with hips and knees extended in a neutral position. The scrotum should be gently supported with paper towel between the thighs. Both testes are examined, the unaffected testis first. The transducer is placed in longitudinal section and transverse section on each testicle in turn. A transverse section to include both testes on one image should be obtained to compare the echogenicity (Fig. 13.3).

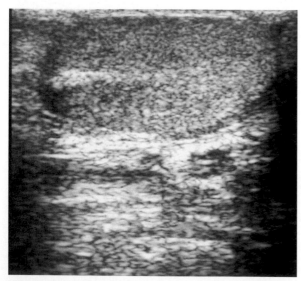

Figure 13.1 — Normal ultrasonic appearances of the testis in longitudinal section. Echogenic line is due to the mediastinum of the testis. Note the thin, echogenic rim which represents the tunica albuginea.

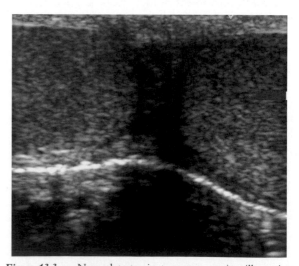

Figure 13.3 — Normal testes in transverse section illustrating equal echogenicity and size.

In infants, the testes can be mobile structures within the scrotum and will need to be gently held and supported in position when scanning.

Assessment and measurement of each testis can be made.

RENAL ASSESSMENT

Complete examination should always include views of the kidneys and bladder.

Cryptoorchidism (undescended)

Incomplete descent of the testis into the scrotum.

Incidence: 3–4% of full term male births increasing to 30% in premature infants. After the age of 1 year only 0.8% of infants will have true cryptoorchidism. The migration of the testis from the posterior abdominal wall into the scrotum can be arrested anywhere along its course. 80–90% of apparently undescended testes will be located in the inguinal canal. 10–20% are located in the abdomen. Cryptoorchidism can be bilateral.

CLINICAL PRESENTATION

Non palpable testis.

TECHNIQUE

As the vast majority will be located in the inguinal canal, the ultrasound examination should include this area.

ULTRASOUND APPEARANCES

- The undescended testis appears elliptical in shape with uniform medium level echoes.

- An inguinal testis may be smaller in size than normal, may be dysplastic and appear hypoechoic (Fig. 13.4).

TREATMENT

Surgical correction (orchidopexy) by the age of 2 years is necessary to preserve fertility and prevent malignancy if the testis remains undescended.

PITFALLS

A lymph node or a gubernaculum testis can be mistaken for a small, dysplastic inguinal testis.

LIMITATIONS

An ectopic testis, that is in the abdomen or pelvis, is difficult to locate. Further evaluation is with MRI or

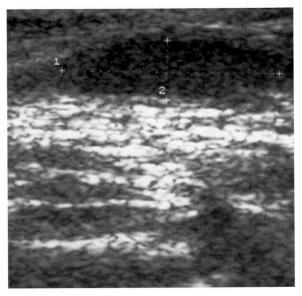

Figure 13.4 — Small right testis located in the inguinal canal. When ectopic the testis does not demonstrate the normal structures such as the epididymis and mediastinum due to compression.

laparoscopy. If the ipsilateral kidney is absent, then the testis is also absent.

MERITS

Location of the ectopic testis by ultrasonic methods assists management.

ASSOCIATED ANOMALIES

Urological anomalies such as duplex systems, renal agenesis, renal malrotation, hypoplasia.

Prune belly syndrome.

Imperforate anus.

Noonan syndrome.

Intersex.

Hydrocele

A collection of fluid surrounding the testis.

May be congenital or acquired.

Acquired lesions are secondary to inflammation, trauma, torsion or neoplasms.

The most common cause of a scrotal mass.

Can be unilateral or bilateral.

CLINICAL PRESENTATION

Swollen scrotum.

TECHNIQUE

Axial and sagittal scans of the whole scrotum and both testes must be done. Great care and gentleness are required whilst scanning if the scrotum is inflamed or trauma has occurred.

ULTRASOUND APPEARANCES

- The testis is surrounded by an anechoic fluid collection which should be unilocular (Fig. 13.5).

- A multiloculated collection suggests infection, haemorrhage or tumour (Fig. 13.6).

- In traumatic or infected hydroceles there is often debris in the fluid (Fig. 13.7).

- Chronic hydroceles can be associated with scrotal wall thickening over 6 mm.

TREATMENT

Antibiotics are given if the lesion is traumatic or infective. Surgery may be required for large lesions.

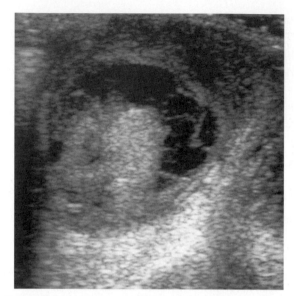

Figure 13.6 — A multiloculated infected hydrocele.

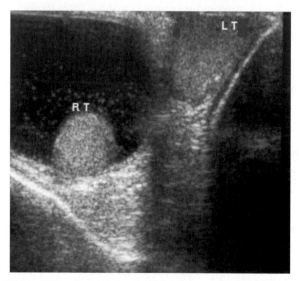

Figure 13.7 — Large hydrocele with echogenic debris within the fluid due to infection.

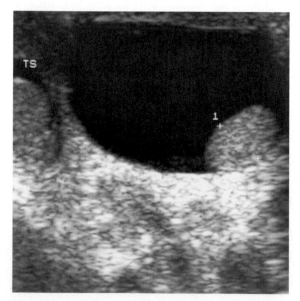

Figure 13.5 — One-month-old child showing a large, simple hydrocele surrounding a normal volume testis.

MERITS

High sensitivity of ultrasound in detecting hydroceles.

Epididymitis/Epididymoorchitis

Inflammation of the epididymis due to infection.

Mostly idiopathic.

Known association: mumps and TB.

CLINICAL PRESENTATION

Swollen, sore testis and hemiscrotum.

Fever and pyuria.

ULTRASOUND TECHNIQUE

In addition to standard greyscale imaging, colour flow imaging should be used to demonstrate the typically increased blood flow to the epididymis and testis.

ULTRASOUND APPEARANCES

- Enlarged epididymis with decreased echogenicity (Fig. 13.8).

- If there is epididymoorchitis there is enlargement of the testis with focal or generalised decreased echogenicity of both it and the epididymis.

- Increased blood flow to the epididymis and testis is seen with colour flow (Fig. 13.9). A small reactive hydrocele may be present.

TREATMENT

Antibiotics.

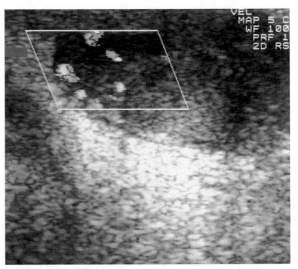

Figure 13.9 — Colour flow shows increased vascularity of the epididymis due to infection.

PITFALLS

A complication of epididymitis/epididymoorchitis is testicular ischaemia which occurs when the enlarged epididymis or oedematous spermatic cord compresses the spermatic vessels.

The testis is enlarged and heterogeneous and has decreased or absent colour flow.

LIMITATIONS

Assessment of blood flow may be impossible due to movement of the patient (movement artefact).

MERITS

Accurate diagnosis will prevent surgical scrotal exploration. The main differential diagnosis is testicular torsion which needs urgent surgery. If there is any doubt about the ultrasonic diagnosis, surgical exploration is indicated.

Torsion

Axial twisting of the spermatic cord about itself, obstructing blood flow and leading to testicular necrosis.

AGE RANGE

Mostly between ages 12 and 18 years due to rapid growth of the genitalia, but may occur at any age, even antenatally.

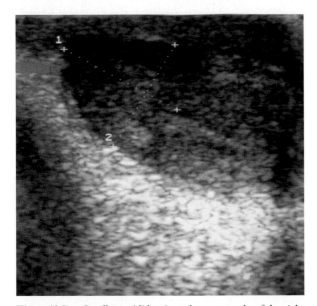

Figure 13.8 — Swollen epididymis at the upper pole of the right testis due to epididymitis.

CLINICAL PRESENTATION

Sudden acute onset of pain.

Nausea and vomiting.

Smooth firm scrotal mass; the testis may have a transverse lie.

Discoloured tender scrotum.

TECHNIQUE

In addition to standard real time grey scale ultrasound, colour flow imaging should be used to demonstrate absence of blood flow in the affected testis. Careful setting of colour flow parameters is needed as the velocity of blood flow within the small testicular vessels is low. If the colour velocity range is set too high then low velocity blood flow will not be detected. The colour gain should be increased just until background noise is visible (Fig. 13.10).

ULTRASOUND APPEARANCES

This is dependent on the time elapsed since onset of symptoms.

- Initially the testicular architecture is normal.

- After 4–6 hours the testis is enlarged with decreased echogenicity compared with the normal contralateral testis due to oedema. The epididymis is enlarged and hypoechoic due to impaired blood supply.

- After 24 hours the testis becomes heterogeneous due to necrosis and haemorrhage.

- A reactive hydrocoele may be present and there may be scrotal wall thickening.

- No vascular flow is detected in the testis.

- Flow within the scrotal wall as a result of reactive hyperaemia can be seen on colour flow imaging (Fig. 13.11).

TREATMENT

Surgery – immediate detorsion, fixation of the testis to the scrotal wall and contralateral orchidopexy if the testis is salvageable.

PITFALLS

With infants it can be difficult to demonstrate blood flow as the testes are small and the ultrasound machine may not be sensitive enough to be sure of a diagnosis of torsion. If unsure, surgical exploration is indicated. The differential diagnosis is epididymo-orchitis. The two conditions cannot be distinguished without colour flow imaging.

Appendicular torsion

Axial twisting of the appendix testis which is a vestigial remnant of the Müllerian duct and is attached to the upper pole of the testis by a small stalk.

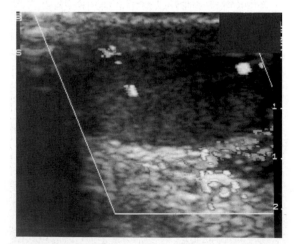

Figure 13.10 — Normal blood flow in the testis. It is normal to find a few colour flashes.

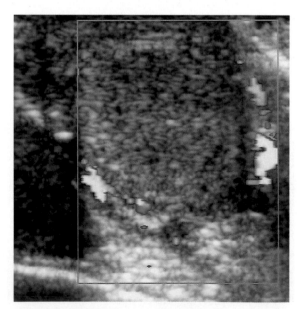

Figure 13.11 — Torsion of testis. There is absence of blood flow on colour imaging with increased blood flow in the scrotal wall.

AGE RANGE

6–12 years but most often in pre-adolescent boys.

CLINICAL PRESENTATION

Acute pain usually localised to the upper pole of the testis.

Small, firm paratesticular nodule with a bluish discoloration.

TECHNIQUE

In addition to standard grey scale imaging, colour flow imaging may demonstrate increased peritesticular blood flow.

ULTRASOUND APPEARANCES

- Normally the appendix testis is not seen but with torsion and inflammation it may be identified and appears as a small hyper/hypoechoic mass at the upper pole of the testis.
- A reactive hydrocele may be present.
- Colour flow will show normal vascularity of the testis with a hypervascular periphery to the mass adjacent to the testis.

TREATMENT

Surgery may be needed to excise the torted appendix. Torsion of the appendicular testis is an isolated lesion and is not normally associated with torsion of the whole organ.

Varicocele

Acquired dilatation of the pampiniform venous plexus of the spermatic cord.

Most occur on the left although they can be bilateral. Idiopathic varicoceles result from incompetent valves in the testicular veins, allowing retrograde flow into the pampiniform venous plexus. It is thought that varicoceles cause infertility because they are associated with low sperm counts and decreased spermatic motility.

CLINICAL PRESENTATION

Enlarged testis with distended veins.

TECHNIQUE

Colour flow and Doppler imaging are necessary for evaluation of the venous problem. The testis must also be routinely assessed. The patient should be scanned

standing and also when performing the Valsalva manoeuvre as the varicocele will increase in size. A compressive mass in the pelvis can also cause a varicocele. The pelvis should always be examined.

ULTRASOUND APPEARANCES

- The veins appear as tortuous, hypoechoic structures with venous flow on Doppler studies (Figs. 13.12, 13.13).

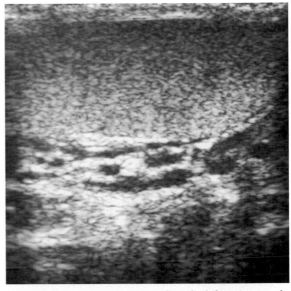

Figure 13.12 — Varicocele surrounding the left testis; note the normal testis. The tubular, hypoechoic structures posterior to the testis are the varicocele veins.

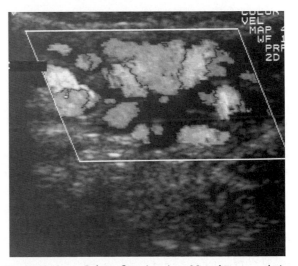

Figure 13.13 — Colour flow imaging. Note hypervascularity within varicocele veins.

- They can measure between 2 and 7 mm in diameter (the diameter of a normal vein measures 0.5–2 mm).

- The varicocele increases in size when the patient is standing or performing the Valsalva manoeuvre.

TREATMENT

The preferred treatment is by embolisation with insertion of platinum spirals into the testicular vein and at the insertion of collaterals to occlude the blood flow from the varicocele. Surgical ligation of the feeding veins is an alternative treatment. Treatment does not cause testicular infarction.

PITFALL

If the varicocele is associated with an arteriovenous malformation then embolisation may not be the preferred treatment option. Full mapping of the arteriovenous malformation is required.

Epididymal cyst/spermatocele

Cystic dilatation of the efferent tubules of the epididymis.

Usually secondary to trauma or chronic epididymitis, most spermatoceles are located near the upper pole of the testis or in the head of the epididymis. Epididymal cysts can occur anywhere along the course of the epididymis.

CLINICAL PRESENTATION

Swelling of the epididymis in the hemiscrotum.

TECHNIQUE

The head of the epididymis is located adjacent to the superior pole of the testis at its posterolateral aspect. The transducer position is altered slowly in longitudinal section until the swollen epididymal head is seen, and measurements can be made.

ULTRASOUND APPEARANCES

- An epididymal cyst and a spermatocele both appear as an anechoic or hypoechoic fluid filled structure.

- They both have thin walls and acoustic enhancement (Fig. 13.14).

TREATMENT

Antibiotics.

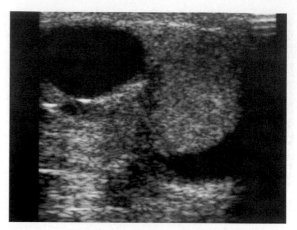

Figure 13.14 — Typical appearances of an epididymal cyst within the epididymis. Small hydrocele is also present.

MERITS

High sensitivity of ultrasound in detecting cysts.

Tumour

The most common type is infantile embryonal cell cancer and can occur in both normally positioned and undescended testes. The second most frequent are non-germ cell tumours such as rhabdomyosarcomas and constitute approximately 24% of testicular tumours in prepubertal children. Testicular infiltration by metastases, leukaemia and lymphoma also occurs.

CLINICAL PRESENTATION

Painless, unilateral, firm testicular enlargement.

TECHNIQUE

The examination should include assessment of the pelvic and para-aortic nodes, and the liver.

ULTRASOUND APPEARANCES

- Variable appearances.

- They can be well defined or diffuse (Fig. 13.15) with variable echogenicity ranging from hypo to hyperechoic.

- The parenchyma can be homogeneous or heterogeneous with areas of decreased echogenicity due to necrosis, haemorrhage or cysts, or with areas of increased echogenicity due to fat or calcification.

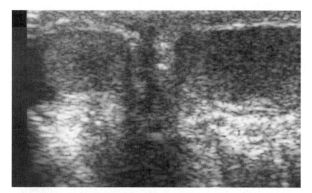

Figure 13.15 — Lymphomatous infiltration of the left testis. Note enlargement relative to the right. In this case, no discrete tumour.

- It is impossible to tissue type a neoplastic testicular mass due to the significant overlap in ultrasonic appearances. Biopsy is required for diagnosis.

- There may be a reactive hydrocele.

- On colour flow imaging the vascularity of the tumour varies with its size.

- Small tumours tend to be avascular and larger tumours are often hypervascular.

TREATMENT
Surgery and chemotherapy.

Acute scrotal oedema

CLINICAL PRESENTATION
Sudden onset of painful, swollen scrotum.

May extend to the inguinal region.

Cause unknown

AGE RANGE:
Mostly between the ages: 4 and 7 years.

ULTRASOUND APPEARANCES
- Thickening and oedema of scrotal wall.

- May be an associated hydrocele.

- Underlying testis and epididymis are normal.

- On colour imaging the testicular flow remains normal. There can be increased flow in the scrotal wall (Fig. 13.16).

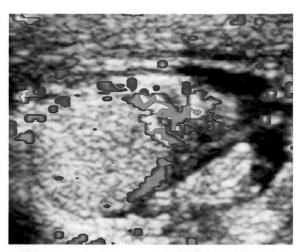

Figure 13.16 — Idiopathic scrotal oedema in a four-year-old showing normal flow within the testis and increased flow in the scrotal wall.

TREATMENT
Resolves spontaneously within several days.

Scrotal trauma

CLINICAL PRESENTATION
Painful, swollen, discoloured scrotum following direct trauma.

ULTRASOUND APPEARANCES
- Thickening of scrotal wall.

- Echogenic fluid around the testes due to haemorrhage if acute.

- Echogenic focus in the testes due to haemorrhage.

- Fracture of the testis may occur.

Appearances of a haematoma/haematocele can be varied, depending on their age, from increased to decreased echogenicity; they become complex in appearance as the blood liquefies (Fig. 13.17).

TREATMENT
Surgery is required within the first 72 hours to salvage a ruptured testis.

Fracture, small haematomas and haematoceles are not indications for surgery as long as the tunica albuginea is intact and blood flow to the testis is preserved. Large torsion haematoceles may require aspiration as they can compress the testis, causing ischaemia.

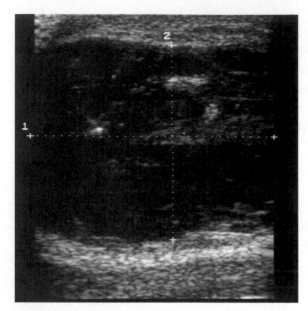

Figure 13.17 — An extratesticular haematocele of the left scrotum several days following direct injury. It is a complex mass with anechoic areas and septations as the blood liquefies.

Further reading

Atkinson GO Jr, Patrick LE, Ball TI Jr, Stephenson CA, Broecker BH, Woodward JR. The normal and abnormal scrotum in children: evaluation with color Doppler sonography. *AJR* 1992; **158**: 613–617.

Bird K, Rosenfield AT, Taylor KJW. Ultrasonography in testicular torsion. *Radiology* 1983; **147**: 527–534.

Burks DD, Markey BJ, Burkhard TK, Balsara ZN, Haluszka MM, Canning DA. Suspected testicular torsion and ischemia: evaluation with color Doppler sonography. *Radiology* 1990; **175**: 815–821.

Fakhry J, Khoury A, Barakat K. The hypoechoic band: a normal finding on testicular sonography. *AJR* 1989; **153**: 321–323.

Friedland GW, Chang P. The role of imaging in the management of the impalpable undescended testis. *AJR* 1988; **151**: 1107–1111.

Horstman WG, Melson GL, Middleton WD, Andriole GL. Testicular tumors: findings with color Doppler US. *Radiology* 1992; **185**: 733–737.

Horstman WG, Middleton WD, Melson GL. Scrotal inflammatory disease: color Doppler US findings. *Radiology* 1991; **179**: 55–59.

Lerner RM, Mevorach RA, Hulbert WC, Rabinowitz R. Color Doppler US in the evaluation of acute scrotal disease. *Radiology* 1990; **176**: 355–358.

Luker GD, Siegel MJ. Pediatric testicular tumors: evaluation with gray scale and color Doppler US. *Radiology* 1994; **191**: 561–564.

Rifkin MD, Foy PM, Kurtz AB, Pasto ME, Goldberg BB. The role of diagnostic ultrasonography in varicocele evaluation. *J Ultrasound Med* 1983; **2**: 271–275.

Rifkin MD, Kurtz AB, Goldberg BB. Epididymis examined by ultrasound. *Radiology* 1984; **151**: 187–190.

Sudakoff GS, Burke M, Rifkin MD. Ultrasonographic and color Doppler imaging of hemorrhagic epididymitis in Henoch-Schönlein purpura. *J Ultrasound Med* 1992; **11**: 619–621.

14

THE MUSCULOSKELETAL SYSTEM

None required.

TRANSDUCER

High frequency – 10 MHz linear transducer; a lower frequency transducer may be required to achieve the depth of penetration for deeper lesions, e.g. in the thigh.

TECHNIQUE

Longitudinal and transverse sections of the area of interest should be performed. Where possible, comparison with the normal contralateral side, examined in the same position, should be made. A dynamic study may be useful, particularly when muscles or tendons are involved. Small muscle tears are more obvious when a muscle contracts. Flexion and extension of tendons whilst scanning will help to diagnose discontinuity or impingement.

Colour flow imaging is essential to demonstrate the vascularity of a lesion and therefore aid in its diagnosis.

For very superficial lesions the use of a stand off may be required.

Normal tissue characteristics

Vary with beam obliquity and transducer frequency.

Tendon

Well-defined, echogenic structure with fine parallel internal echoes. The peritendon sheath appears as a thin echogenic line either side of the tendon (Fig. 14.1).

Muscle

Hypoechoic, with fine parallel echogenic echoes resulting in a feather like appearance (Fig. 14.2).

Ligament

Similar to tendons, with a less regular internal pattern.

Nerves

Echogenic, similar to tendons, although internal echoes are much longer than those seen in tendons.

Adipose

Variable, depending on size of adipocytes. Subcutaneous fat appears hypoechoic and contains thin linear echoes – strands of connective tissue.

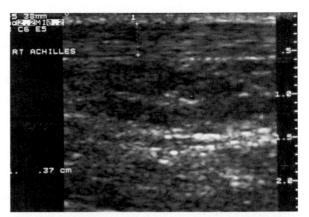

Figure 14.1 — Normal tendon. The normal achilles tendon, a well-defined echogenic structure with fine parallel internal echoes.

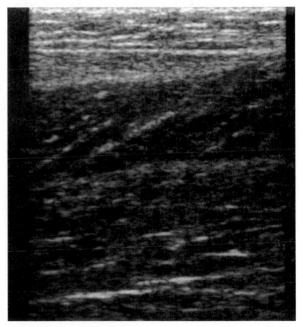

Figure 14.2 — Normal muscle appears hypoechoic with fine parallel echogenic echoes resulting in a featherlike appearance.

Bone

Anterior surface appears echogenic (strongly reflective) with acoustic shadowing posteriorly.

Hyaline cartilage

Articular cartilage appears hypoechoic/anechoic. Echogenicity increases with age (Fig. 14.3).

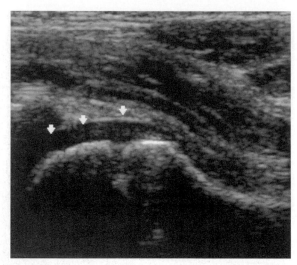

Figure 14.3 — Normal hypoechoic appearance of the hyaline articular cartilage of the femoral head in a 4-year-old child.

FIBRO-CARTILAGE
Homogeneous echogenic structure.

Soft tissue masses

Ultrasound can be used to determine:

- The presence of a mass.
- Its position (masses can occur in skin, fat, muscle, lymph node) and appearance, e.g. cystic/solid, well defined/irregular (well-defined lesions are usually benign, irregular lesions are more often malignant).
- Capsule vascularity.
- ? displaces/invades surrounding tissues.

Malignant

Rhabdomyosarcoma

This is the most common soft tissue sarcoma in children; it occurs in muscle.

CLINICAL PRESENTATION
Variable – symptoms depend on site.

History usually of a rapidly enlarging mass.

Often not very painful.

ULTRASOUND APPEARANCES (Fig. 14.4)
- Variable: hypoechoic – echogenic
- Heterogeneous.
- Irregular walls, although may be well-defined.
- Highly vascular on colour Doppler.

Other malignant soft tissue tumours include fibrosarcomas, synovial sarcomas and malignant schwannomas. All have similar clinical presentation and ultrasound appearances as rhabdomyosarcomas.

Benign

Haemangiomas

A benign vascular tumour. There are two types: capillary and cavernous.

The most common tumours of infancy, and usually absent at birth, they appear during the first month of life, gradually increasing in size until 6–10 months when they tend to stabilise; involution then occurs and by the age of 7 years most have resolved.

CLINICAL PRESENTATION
Palpable mass.

Skin discoloration – may not be present if the lesion is 'deep'.

ULTRASOUND APPEARANCES (Fig. 14.5)
- Capillary haemangiomas – echogenic.

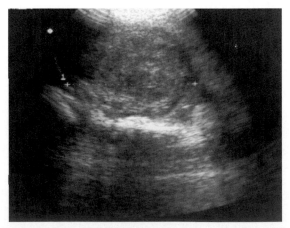

Figure 14.4 — Rhabdomyosarcoma. A heterogeneous well-defined mass in the posterior right thigh.

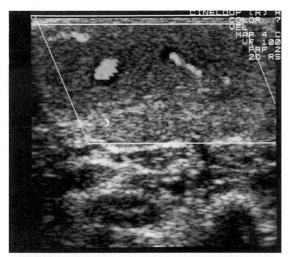

Figure 14.5 — Cavernous haemangioma. A hyperechoic mass in the superficial tissues of the thigh with feeding vessels on colour Doppler.

- Cavernous – complex mass with septations.

  - feeding and draining vessels on colour Doppler.

Full mapping requires MR imaging.

TREATMENT
Only if causing functional or aesthetic problems.

Lymphangioma

A benign tumour of the lymphatic system, variable in size.

SITE
Most frequent in the neck, often called cystic hygromas, they occur in axilla, shoulder girdle, mediastinum and abdomen.

CLINICAL PRESENTATION
Palpable mass.

Pain or sudden enlargement if haemorrhage occurs within the lesion.

ULTRASOUND APPEARANCES (Fig. 14.6)
- Thin-walled multi-locular cystic structures.

- Occasionally occur as solitary cysts.

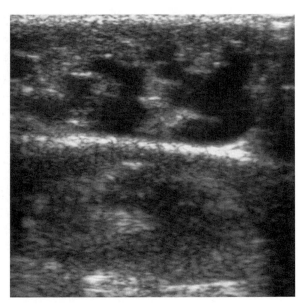

Figure 14.6 — Lymphangioma. A longitudinal section of the left forearm demonstrating a hypoechoic multi-locular mass anterior to the muscle.

- If haemorrhage occurs, become more echogenic and may compress or displace vessels and surrounding structures.

- Ill-defined.

- No obvious blood flow on colour Doppler.

Lipoma

A benign tumour which develops in the fat cells of the subcutaneous tissues.

Usually slow growing, it is not common in children.

CLINICAL PRESENTATION
Slow growing mass

Soft/doughy feel on palpation.

ULTRASOUND APPEARANCES (Fig. 14.7)
- Usually highly echogenic, but may be hypoechoic or isoechoic.

- 'Thinly' encapsulated mass.

- Variable size.

- No blood flow on colour Doppler.

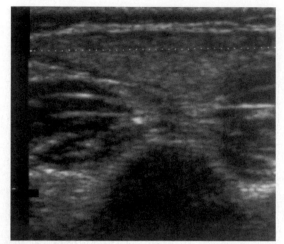

Figure 14.7 — Lipoma. A transverse section of the posterior neck demonstrates a well-defined echogenic mass with a thin wall, the appearances consistent with a lipoma.

Cystic lesions

Ganglion

Cystic swelling which develops in connection with a tendon sheath.

Most commonly occurs at the wrist.

CLINICAL PRESENTATION

Palpable swelling.

Usually painless.

ULTRASOUND APPEARANCES (Fig. 14.8)

- Uni/multi-loculated.
- Well-defined.
- Anechoic.
- Post-cystic enhancement.

Synovial cysts

These develop from joint spaces or adjacent bursae. The most common – popliteal (Baker's) cyst – is a fluid collection in the gastrocnemio semi-membranous bursa.

CLINICAL PRESENTATION OF A POPLITEAL CYST

Asymptomatic mass behind the knee.

Pain.

May be associated with trauma.

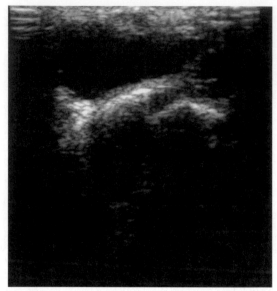

Figure 14.8 — Ganglion. A well-defined anechoic lesion anterior to the carpal bones.

ULTRASOUND APPEARANCES (Fig. 14.9a, b)

- Well-defined cystic collection posterior to the knee, which demonstrates enhancement posteriorly.
- Communication with the joint space is often difficult to demonstrate.
- Debris/septae in infected cysts.
- No blood flow within the lesion on colour flow imaging.
  (Differential diagnosis is an aneurysm of the popliteal artery, which may have a similar presentation but turbulent blood flow will be seen on colour flow and this is very rare in children.)

TREATMENT

No treatment is usually required as they resolve spontaneously.

Meniscal cyst (Fig. 14.10)

A cyst which develops as a result of a meniscal tear.

CLINICAL PRESENTATION

Dull pain at the site of the 'mass' usually worse after exertion.

A mass which is more prominent when the affected joint is extended rather than flexed.

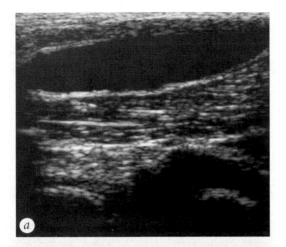

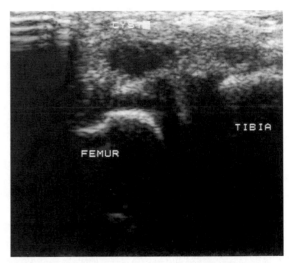

Figure 14.10 — A longitudinal section demonstrating an anechoic area lateral to the knee joint, a meniscal cyst.

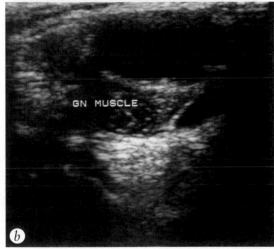

Figure 14.9 — Popliteal cyst (a) A longitudinal section of the popliteal fossa demonstrates a well-defined anechoic lesion posterior to the knee joint. (b) In transverse section, the cystic lesion is shown to extend around the origin of the gastrocnemius medialis muscle.

CLINICAL PRESENTATION

Trauma.

Bleeding disorders, e.g. haemophilia.

ULTRASOUND APPEARANCES (Fig. 14.11a–d)

- Variable, depending on age.
- Fresh clot appears echogenic.
- As liquefaction occurs becomes less echogenic.
- As organisation occurs, septations and internal echoes are seen.
- Well-defined or irregular outline.
- Post-cystic enhancement.

NB. A cephalhaematoma is a haematoma which occurs on the scalp and is a result of birth trauma (Fig. 14.11d). It often does not present initially, and is diagnosed later when a lump is felt on the head.

ULTRASOUND APPEARANCES

- Small well-defined cyst.
- May be multi-locular.
- Often contain internal echoes.
- Post cystic enhancement.

Haematomas

Result from haemorrhage within soft tissues, muscles, tendons.

Soft tissue infections

CLINICAL PRESENTATION

Pain

Fever

Malaise

Erythematous/indurated area on skin.

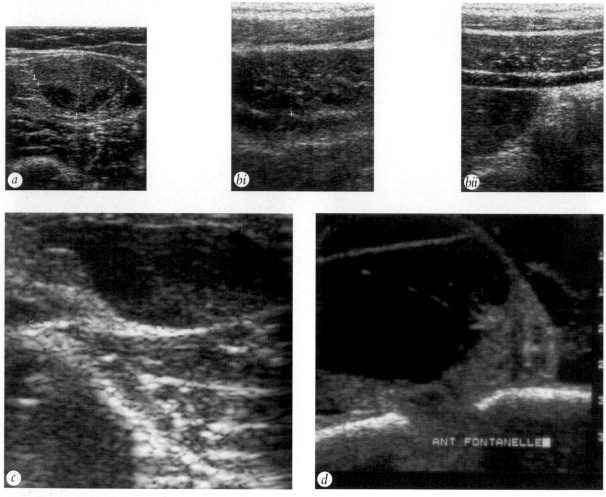

Figure 14.11 — Haematomas. (a) A well-defined heterogeneous mass within the muscle following trauma. (b) Loss of normal echotexture and an increase in depth of the abdominal wall muscle (i), in comparison to the contralateral side (ii), following direct trauma, suggestive of haematoma. (c) A well-defined anechoic lesion with posterior enhancement and some internal echoes, suggestive of a resolving haematoma. (d) An anechoic collection with strands in the soft tissues of the scalp, appearances consistent with a cephalhaematoma.

Abscess

ULTRASOUND APPEARANCES (Fig. 14.12)

- Elliptical/spherical shaped mass.

- Hypoechoic.

- Post-cystic enhancement.

- Echogenic foci with acoustic shadowing indicating the presence of gas forming organisms.

- Hyperaemia at the periphery of the lesion on colour flow imaging.

- May be associated with a foreign body.

PITFALL

May be difficult to differentiate from haematoma or necrotic tumour on ultrasound; clinical presentation will help diagnosis.

TREATMENT

Ultrasound guided aspiration/drainage may be performed.

Cellulitis

Infection of skin and subcutaneous tissues without focal abscess formation. The infected area is hot, red

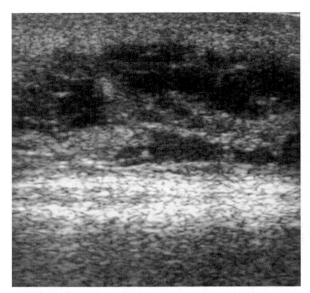

Figure 14.12 — Abscess. A complex mass with irregular walls demonstrating some post-cystic enhancement. Note the oedema of the surrounding tissues.

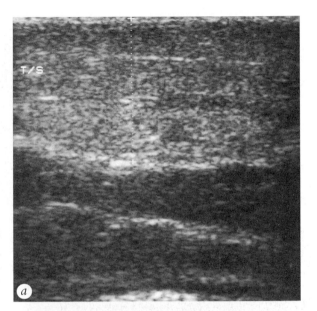

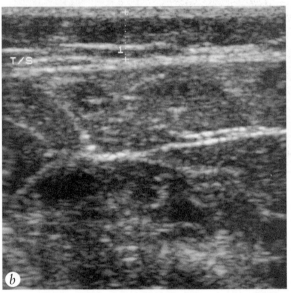

Figure 14.13 — Cellulitis. Diffuse increase in the depth and echogenicity of the soft tissues (a), in comparison to the contralateral side (b), consistent with cellulitis.

and swollen. The child usually has a fever. Cellulitis may reflect underlying osteomyelitis or abscess. Cellulitis is treated with antibiotics. Abscess and osteomyelitis may need surgical drainage.

ULTRASOUND APPEARANCES (Fig. 14.13)

- Thickening of the subcutaneous tissue with increased echogenicity compared with contralateral site.

- Normal muscle unless there is also myositis.

Osteomyelitis

Occurs in all age groups.

Causes include bacilli, fungi, viruses and parasites.

Infection of adjacent soft tissues, surgery, and haematogenous spread are all routes of infection.

CLINICAL PRESENTATION

Pain and swelling.

Reluctance to move affected area.

Fever.

+/– associated cellulitis.

ULTRASOUND APPEARANCES (Fig. 14.14)

- Small fluid collection contiguous with affected bone or within soft tissues.

- +/– soft tissue oedema.

- +/– joint effusion.

- Peripheral flow on colour Doppler.

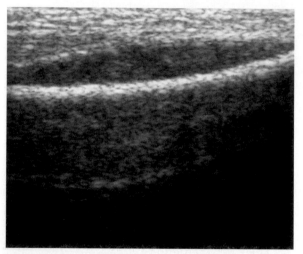

Figure 14.14 — Osteomyelitis. A longitudinal section of the tibia demonstrating a fluid collection contiguous with bone.

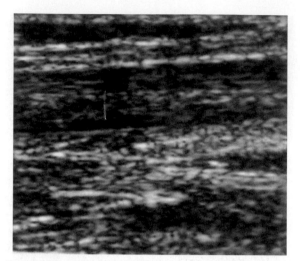

Figure 14.15 — Tendonitis. The tendon appears thickened.

Pyomyositis

Results in oedema and necrosis of muscle.

Rare in non-tropical countries.

ULTRASOUND APPEARANCES
- Enlarged muscle.
- Hypoechoic.
- May contain echogenic debris.
- The presence of gas forming organisms will result in echogenic foci with acoustic shadowing.

Tendonitis

Inflammation of a tendon.

Caused by repetitive use, e.g. sports activities.

May be diffuse or nodular.

CLINICAL PRESENTATION
Pain.

Tendon appears bulky on examination.

ULTRASOUND APPEARANCES (Fig. 14.15)

Acute

- Focal thickening of the tendon associated with an area of decreased echogenicity, which has less well-defined internal echoes.

Chronic

- The tendon appears increased in echogenicity.
- Minute calcifications are often seen as punctate hyperechoic foci with acoustic shadowing.

Trauma

The cause of most pathological conditions which affect muscles and tendons.

Acute injuries in muscles

Result in:

Haematomas – appearances variable depending on age of haematoma – see previously.

Rupture/tear.

ULTRASOUND APPEARANCES
Small tears (Fig. 14.16)
- Discontinuity of muscle fibres or the presence of a haematoma.
- A hypoechoic area within the muscle.
- Dynamic evaluation is essential, contraction demonstrates retraction of muscle with an increase in the size of the lesion if there is a tear.
- A muscle haematoma does not change in size.

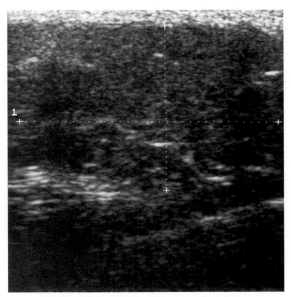

Figure 14.16 — Loss of normal muscle architecture with associated haemorrhage, consistent with a muscle tear.

Large tears

- The retracted muscle is seen surrounded by haematoma to give the classic 'Clapper in the bell' appearance.

- Fibrosis and scarring may develop following large tears which have gone untreated. A hyperechoic irregular area, which does not alter with contraction is seen, sometimes with acoustic shadowing.

Acute injuries in tendons

Result in:

Haematomas – see previously.

Tears.

ULTRASOUND APPEARANCES

- **Partial** (Fig. 14.17)
Focal hypoechoic defect in the body of the tendon or at its attachment.

- **Complete**
Complete disruption of the tendon with variable amounts of retraction of the fragments from one another. There may or may not be associated haematoma. A chronic tear may result in an echogenic fibrous scar.

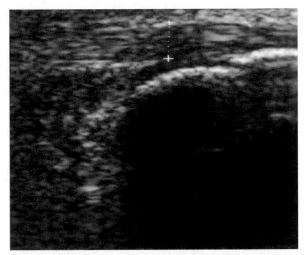

Figure 14.17 — Tendon tear – partial. Note the hypoechoic area just above the insertion of the Achilles in the calcaneum disrupting the normal fine linear striation of the tendon.

Foreign bodies

Wood, glass and metal most commonly encountered, usually in hands and feet.

CLINICAL PRESENTATION

History of injury/penetrating injury.

Pain.

Swelling.

Infection.

ULTRASOUND APPEARANCES (Fig. 14.18)

- Echogenic structure with or without acoustic shadowing.

- +/– granuloma.

Granuloma

Small nodular inflammatory lesion.

Often associated with foreign bodies.

CLINICAL PRESENTATION

Hard lump.

+/– swelling, pain.

ULTRASOUND APPEARANCE (Fig. 14.19)

Well-defined hypoechoic lesion.

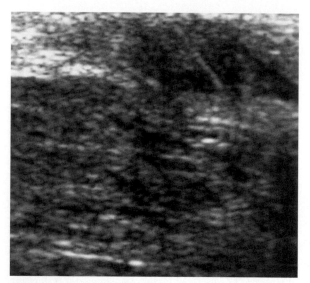

Figure 14.18 — A foreign body is seen as a linear echogenic structure within a well-defined hypoechoic lesion consistent with granuloma formation.

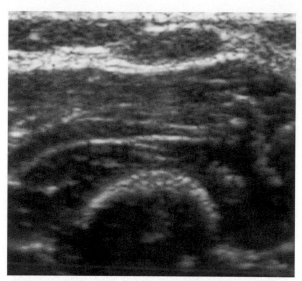

Figure 14.19 — Granuloma. A well-defined hypoechoic lesion within the subcutaneous tissues, anterior to the muscle.

THE HIP

Hip effusion

This is an abnormal collection of fluid within the hip joint caused, most commonly, by synovitis. Other causes include septic arthritis, juvenile rheumatoid arthritis, slipped upper femoral epiphysis and Perthes' disease.

Approximately 50% of children with acute hip pain will have intra-articular fluid.

Age range: 2–10 years.

It is more common in boys.

CLINICAL PRESENTATION

Hip pain.

Limited movement with the leg held in external rotation.

Reluctance to weight bear.

Pyrexia is not normally a feature of idiopathic synovitis but is found in septic arthritis. A mild pyrexia may be present in some children with synovitis as the hip effusion represents a toxic reaction.

CHOICE OF TRANSDUCER

10 MHz linear (7.5 is adequate).

PATIENT PREPARATION

None.

TECHNIQUE

The patient lies supine with the hip and knees extended in a comfortable position. In older boys who may be embarrassed, the genitals should be covered by a towel placed between the legs. Both hips are examined, the unaffected hip first, but held in the same position as the affected hip. The transducer is placed in longitudinal section anteriorly in the groin. Slight rotational movements are needed to obtain a parasagittal image anterior and parallel to the femoral head, neck and shaft (Fig. 14.20). The distance between the outer edge of the femoral neck and the inner edge of the joint capsule in a normal hip is up to 3 mm (Fig. 14.21). More than 2 mm difference between the two hips is regarded as a significant effusion. Transverse sections, with the transducer rotated through 90°, should also be performed as fluid can be demonstrated in recesses not seen on sagittal section.

Bilateral hip effusions are rare.

ULTRASOUND APPEARANCES

- The femoral head, physeal plate, femoral neck and shaft of femur can be recognised as bright echogenic features with distal acoustic shadowing, although

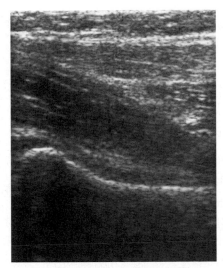

Figure 14.20 — Normal hip joint. The parasagittal image shows the concave joint capsule anterior and parallel to the femoral head, neck and shaft.

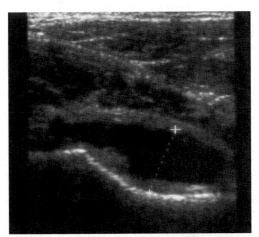

Figure 14.22 — Anechoic hip joint effusion. Note the convex configuration of the joint capsule. The synovium is thickened.

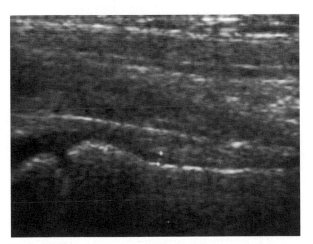

Figure 14.21 — Measurement of the normal joint capsule is up to 3 mm.

the physeal plate formed of cartilage is less echogenic.

- The echogenic joint capsule and hypoechoic ilio-psoas muscle and tendon can be seen anteriorly.
- Fluid accumulates in the joint displacing the joint capsule anteriorly. The joint capsule assumes a convex instead of concave configuration (Fig. 14.22).
- The appearance of the effusion will vary from anechoic to echogenic depending on the composition of the fluid.
- An echogenic effusion is due to haemorrhage or pus.

NB. Most septic effusions are not echogenic and appear as a transonic collection. Thickened synovium may also be seen (Fig. 14.22).

TREATMENT
Aspiration may be required if the effusion is over 5 mm in depth.

PITFALLS
An echogenic effusion may be mistaken for the ileo-psoas muscle.

LIMITATIONS
Patient size may compromise the examination as depth of penetration may be limited.

MERITS
The sensitivity for detection of effusion is over 90%.

ASSOCIATED DISEASE
Occasionally fragmentation of the femoral capital epiphysis in Perthes' disease may be seen, or the step in the epiphyseal plate due to a slipped upper femoral capital epiphysis.

Hip aspiration

Fluid is aspirated from the joint using an aseptic technique under ultrasound control. This alleviates pain. The fluid is sent to Microbiology.

PATIENT PREPARATION

Patient is nil by mouth for 3 hours if analgesic sedation is needed.

Consent form is obtained.

Topical anaesthetic cream is applied over the skin at the proposed puncture site, which should avoid major blood vessels, 30 minutes before the procedure.

CHOICE OF TRANSDUCER

10 MHz linear transducer.

PATIENT POSITION

The procedure is performed with the patient in a supine position.

TECHNIQUE

Anaesthetic cream is removed and the skin wiped clean. The patient is rescanned. The depth of fluid from the skin surface to the middle of the fluid pool is measured. Aspiration may be performed either under direct ultrasound guidance or by premarking of the puncture site following scanning in the longitudinal and transverse planes.

The patient's skin is cleaned with an antiseptic solution. Aspiration is performed using a 20 G needle. A longer needle such as a lumbar puncture needle may be required to pierce the joint capsule in older patients.

The aspirate is placed in a sterile specimen bottle labelled with the patient's details and sent for bacteriological examination.

Congenital dysplasia of the hip

Age range: 2 weeks to 6 months.

Girls are affected 6–8 times as often as boys.

Incidence: 1 in 100 to 1.5 in 1000 neonates.

Risk factors: a family history, breech delivery.

Anatomy

The normal acetabular cartilage complex is a 3-D structure with a tri-radiate cartilage forming the medial border and the cup-shaped acetabular cartilage forming the outer two-thirds of the cavity. When the femoral head is not seated in the acetabulum, the latter becomes dysplastic. Subsequently, the capsule and ligaments stretch; fibrous and fatty tissue develops in the acetabulum and femoral head ossification is delayed.

CLINICAL PRESENTATION

A 'click' is heard on clinical examination (Barlow and Ortolani techniques).

There may be:

Abnormal ligamentous laxity of the hip joint.

Unequal leg length.

Limitation of abduction.

Unequal skin creases.

CHOICE OF TRANSDUCER

10 MHz linear (7.5 adequate).

PATIENT PREPARATION

None.

TECHNIQUE

Two main techniques have developed for evaluating the infant hip; the static scan as proposed by Graf and the dynamic scan as proposed by Harke. The static Graf technique will be described here.

Both hips are examined, the unaffected first. The patient is examined in the lateral decubitus position with the hips and knees flexed to approximately 90 degrees. The transducer is placed lateral to the femur. The hip joint is imaged in coronal section. The position of the femoral head, cartilaginous labrum and the shape of the bony acetabulum are initially subjectively assessed.

Measurements are made of the depth of the bony acetabulum and the position of the labrum so that calculation of the alpha and beta angles can be made.

The dysplastic hip can be classified as unstable with varying degrees of acetabular dysplasia, subluxed, or dislocated (see Table 14.1).

Three lines and two angles are calculated on the image (Figs. 14.23, 14.24):

Line 1 parallels the ilium (baseline).

Line 2 is drawn along the inner edge of the labrum.

Line 3 is drawn along the inner edge of the acetabulum to the tri-radiate cartilage.

Table 14.1 Sonographic classification of hip dysplasia

Type	Alpha angle	Beta angle	Comment
I	> 60	–	Normal
IIA	50–59	–	Physiological immaturity; < 3 months old
IIB	50–59	–	Delayed ossification; > 3 months old
IIC	43–49	< 77	Critical zone; labrum not everted
IID	43–49	> 77	Subluxed; labrum everted
III	< 43	>77	Dislocated
IV	< 43	> 77	Dislocated with labrum interposed between femoral head and acetabulum

Ref: Graf R, Schuler P. *Sonography of the Infant Hip: An atlas.* Germany: VCH, 1986.

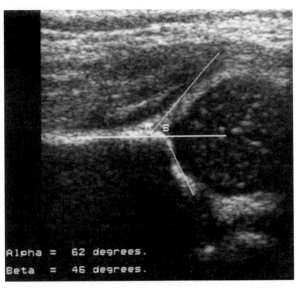

Alpha = 62 degrees.
Beta = 46 degrees.

Figure 14.24 — Corresponding ultrasound image of a normal hip, Graf type I.

The alpha angle = the angle between lines 1 and 3.

The beta angle = the angle between lines 1 and 2.

The smaller the alpha angle and the larger the beta angle are, the more likely that dysplasia is present.

In the Graf technique, there are 4 basic hip types (Fig. 14.25).

Type 1 is normal and requires no follow-up treatment.

Type 2 needs to be closely observed clinically.

Types 3 and 4 require immediate treatment.

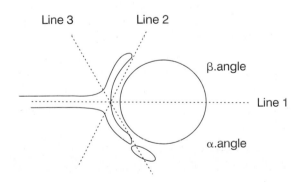

Line 3   Line 2

β.angle

Line 1

α.angle

Figure 14.23 — Line diagram illustrating the three lines needed to calculate the alpha and beta angles.

ULTRASOUND APPEARANCES

Normal

- Ilium – echogenic.

- Ossified portion of the acetabulum – echogenic and casts an acoustic shadow.

- Triradiate cartilage – hypoechoic as it is not ossified and allows sound transmission.

- Femoral head – hypoechoic with fine stippled echoes. At least 50% of the femoral head should lie inferiorly to the baseline.

- Ossification centre – echogenic central area within the femoral head.

- Labrum – echogenic (Fig. 14.26).

Varying degrees of dysplasia can occur with the acetabulum becoming shallower (Figs. 14.27, 14.28). In dislocation the femoral head is usually displaced anteriorly, laterally and superiorly (Fig. 14.29).

TREATMENT

If deemed suitable, an infant with hip dysplasia is treated with a flexion-abduction-external rotation harness (Pavlik) or spica cast. A normal relationship of the acetabulum and femoral head is usually obtained within 6 weeks of treatment.

TYPE I

TYPE II

TYPE III

TYPE IV

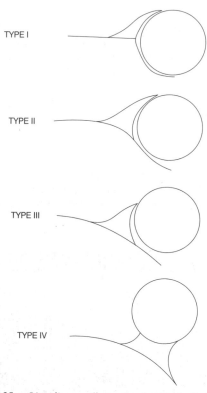

Figure 14.25 — Line diagram illustrating the 4 basic Graf types.

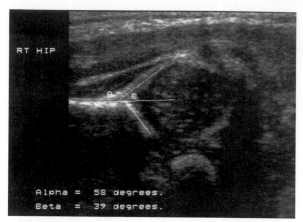

Figure 14.27 — Physiologically immature hip. Infant is less than 3 months of age (Graf type IIA).

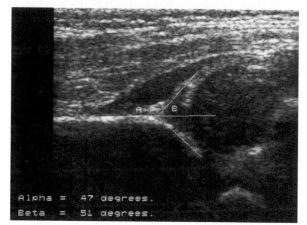

Figure 14.28 — The acetabulum is shallow and the hip is classified as a Graf type IIC.

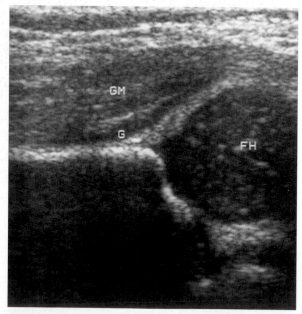

Figure 14.26 — Normal sonographic anatomy of the hip; femoral head (FH), ilium, labrum, tri-radiate cartilage, gluteal muscles (GM: gluteus medius. G: gluteus minimus).

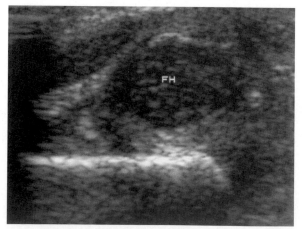

Figure 14.29 — Dislocated hip (Graf type III). The coronal section shows the femoral head (FH) displaced superiorly and laterally out of the acetabulum onto the ilium.

PITFALLS

The ilium must be imaged until it appears horizontal and the maximum depth of the acetabulum obtained. If too anterior or too posterior, then the ilium will not be horizontal but appear curved (Fig. 14.30). The ultrasound machine needs to have a software package enabling the alpha and beta angles to be calculated. While measurements could be made manually post processing of ultrasound film, the software makes it easier.

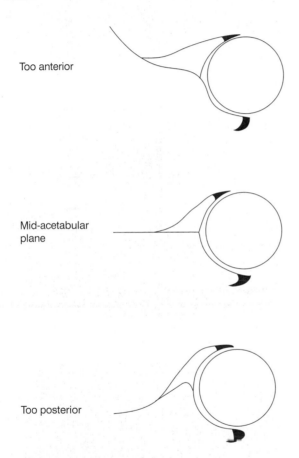

Too anterior

Mid-acetabular
plane

Too posterior

Figure 14.30 — Line diagram illustrating appearances of the ilium too anterior and too posterior to the mid-acetabular plane.

LIMITATIONS

The femoral head begins to ossify at approximately 3 months of age (Fig. 14.31). After 6 months of age the femoral head has ossified sufficiently, preventing accurate measurements to be made due to acoustic shadowing. There is greater depth of fat and gluteal muscles overlying the hips. Monitoring is by radiographs once this occurs.

MERITS

The unossified hip and labrum are clearly demonstrated and a diagnosis of hip dysplasia can be made early. Treatment is more successful if instituted promptly.

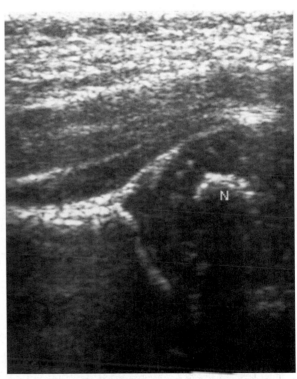

Figure 14.31 — Ossification centre (nucleus – N) of the femoral head in a 4-month-old boy. Note the acoustic shadowing.

THE SPINE

PREPARATION
None required.

TRANSDUCER
High frequency linear transducer, ideally 10 Mhz.

TECHNIQUE
Performed in infants 0–12 months, i.e. before the spinous processes have ossified.

The patient is prone. A foam pad can be placed under the chest and abdomen in infants under 6 months old to try to separate the spinous processes. Assessment is made in sequential longitudinal and transverse sections. To identify the level at which you are scanning either count the vertebrae upwards from the sacral area or use the ribs (tip of last rib – L2) or iliac crest (L4) as landmarks.

Normal ultrasound appearances

In longitudinal section

The spinal cord appears hypo-echoic. Three echogenic lines are seen in parallel representing anterior and posterior walls of the spinal cord and a central echogenic line the central canal. The cord is surrounded by CSF which appears anechoic (Fig. 14.32).

In transverse section

The spinal cord appears oval/round (Fig. 14.33).

Its width varies, the thoracic section being slightly narrower than the cervical and lumbar regions.

It tapers normally at the level of the first and second lumbar vertebrae, the conus medullaris. The tip is called the filum terminale. This extends to the sacral region as a thin echogenic extension of the cord. Filling the cord in this area are echogenic lines, nerve fibres, which almost fill the arachnoid space and can be seen to move on real-time imaging and form the cauda equina.

Tethered cord

Termination of the cord lower than normal, i.e. below L2 (Fig. 14.34).

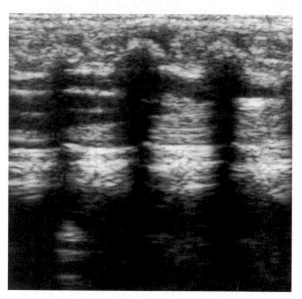

Figure 14.32 — The normal conus medullaris in longitudinal section. The hypoechoic cord with its echogenic walls and central canal is demonstrated tapering to form the conus. Beyond this, the cauda equina is seen as fine echogenic lines.

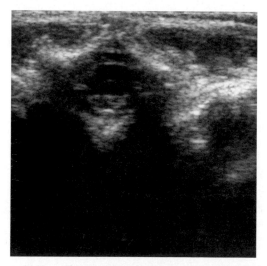

Figure 14.33 — The normal cord appears as an oval hypoechoic structure with the echogenic central canal.

CLINICAL PRESENTATION
Hairy dimple over sacral area, pilonidal sinus or discharging sinus.

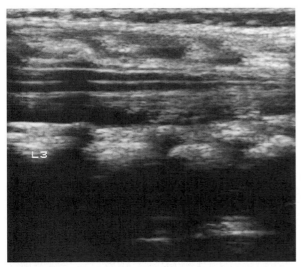

Figure 14.34 — Tethered Cord. The cord is seen extending beyond the L3 and fixed to the posterior wall.

ULTRASOUND APPEARANCES
- Cord extends beyond L1/L2.
- Thickened filum terminale.
- Cord is fixed to the posterior wall.
- Absence of movement of the nerve roots in the cauda equina.

Sacral dimple

CLINICAL PRESENTATION

Small dimple over the sacral area which may have a discharge. Increased risk of meningeal infection if there is a fistula from the skin surface to the spinal canal.

Therefore early diagnosis is important.

ULTRASOUND APPEARANCES
- Hypoechoic track extending from the dimple into the subcutaneous soft tissues, not usually traced to the spinal cord.

ASSOCIATED ANOMALIES

Tethered cord.

Diastematomyelia

This is rare. The cord is split and fixed in position by a bony or fibrous spur extending from the vertebral body.

It is more common in lower thoracic and lumbar regions.

Early diagnosis is essential. Ascent of the cord is prevented by the spur, causing stretching of the cord and the cerebellum and medulla are displaced caudally.

ULTRASOUND APPEARANCES
- Best imaged in transverse section.
- Two round/ovoid cords are seen either side of a bony spur, which appears echogenic.

Diplomyelia

The cord develops as two structures but unlike diastematomyelia has no central bar (Fig. 14.35). It is very rare.

ULTRASOUND APPEARANCES
- Best imaged in transverse section.
- Two cords are seen separated by CSF.

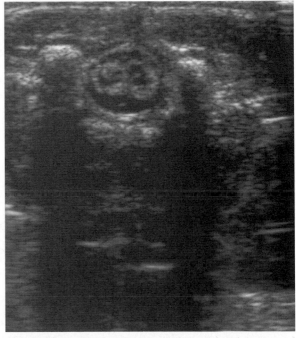

Figure 14.35 — Diplomyelia. Two oval chords are demonstrated in transverse section.

Spinal dysraphism

Meningocele

Cystic congenital herniation of spinal meninges through a defect that does not contain neural tissue.

Myelomeningocele

The herniation contains a component of neural tissue. Often associated with Chiari malformation.

Both usually occur below the second lumbar vertebra, but may also be cervical or thoracic in location.

CLINICAL PRESENTATION

At birth either following antenatal screening or initial paediatric assessment.

ULTRASOUND APPEARANCES

Meningocele (Fig. 14.36)
- Cystic mass in the subcutaneous tissues.
- Cystic element can be demonstrated to be continuous with the spinal canal through a bony defect.

Myelomeningocele
- Cord ends below L2, is tethered and there is loss of movement of the cord.
- Abnormal cord may be herniated into the sac.
- Sac may contain fibrous strands.
- Fibrous strands can be difficult to distinguish from nerve roots; the latter show pulsation on real-time imaging.

Lipomeningocele

Appearance of the cord is similar to myelomeningocele but a fatty/fibrous mass is present in the defect usually with fat in the sacral canal and tethering of the cord.

Syrinx

A cystic fluid-filled space in the cord (Fig. 14.37), most frequent in the cervical cord and associated with a Chiari malformation in most cases.

NB. For most spinal cord abnormalities, MR will be required for full mapping.

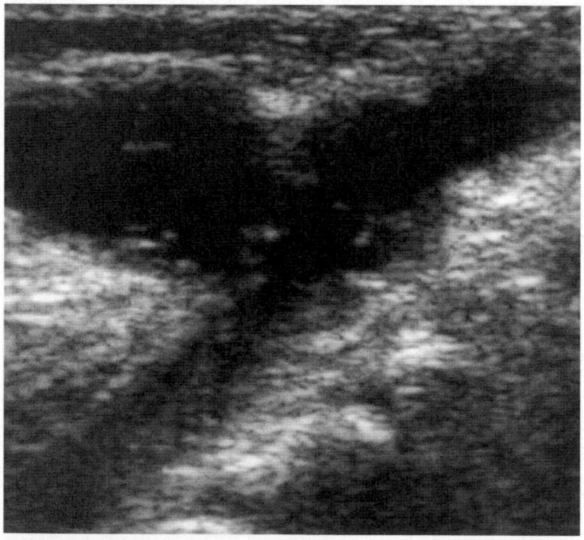

Figure 14.36 — Meningocele a cystic area is demonstrated in the subcutaneous tissues of the sacral region which communicates with the spinal canal.

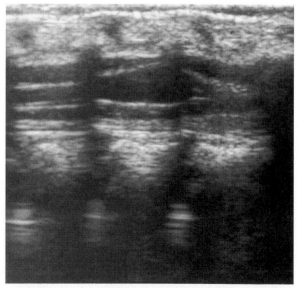

Figure 14.37 — Syrinx a cystic lesion is seen within the spinal cord.

Further reading

Abiri MM, Kirpekar M, Ablow RS Osteomyelitis: detection with US. *Radiology* 1989; **172**: 509–511.

Bertolotto M, Perrone R, Martinoli C et al. High resolution ultrasound anatomy of normal Achilles tendon. *Br J Radiol* 1995; **68**: 986–991.

Breidahl WH, Newman JS, Taljanovic MS et al. Power Doppler sonography in the assessment of musculoskeletal fluid collections. *AJR* 1996; **166**: 1443–1446.

Cardinal E, Buckwalter KA, Braunstein EM, Mih AD. Occult dorsal carpal ganglion: comparison of US and MR imaging. *Radiology* 1994; **193**: 259–262.

Fornage BD. Achilles tendon: US examiation. *Radiology* 1986; **159**: 759–764.

Fornage BD. The hypoechoic normal tendon: a pitfall. *J Ultrasound Med* 1987; **6**: 19–22.

Fornage BD. Ultrasound of the tendons. In: Cosgrove DO, Meire HB, Dewbury KC (eds): *Abdominal and General Ultrasound. Vol 2.* London: Churchill Livingstone, 1993.

Fornage BD, Schernberg FL. Sonographic diagnosis of foreign bodies of the distal extremities. *AJR* 1986; **147**: 567–569.

Fornage BD, Tassin G. Sonographic appearances of superficial soft-tissue lipomas. *JCU* 1991; **19**: 215–220.

Gibbon WW *Musculoskeletal Ultrasound: The essentials.* Greenwich Medical Media, London, 1996.

Gooding GAW, Hardiman T, Sumers M et al. Sonography of the hand and foot in foreign body detection. *J Ultrasound Med* 1987; **6**: 441–447.

Harcke HT, Grissom LE, Finkelstein MS. Evaluation of the musculoskeletal system with sonography. *AJR* 1988; **150**: 1253–1261.

Johnstone AJ, Beggs I. Ultrasound imaging of soft-tissue masses in the extremities. *J Bone Joint Surg* (Br) 1994; **76**B: 688–689.

Kainberger FM, Engel A, Barton P et al. Injury of the Achilles tendon: diagnosis with sonography. *AJR* **155**: 1031–1036.

Kaplan PA, Matamoros A, Anderson JC. sonography of the musculoskeletal system. *AJR* 1990; **155**: 237–245.

Loyer EM, DuBrow RA, David CL et al. Imaging of superficial soft-tissue infections: sonographic findings in cases of cellulitis and abscess. *AJR* 1996; **166**: 149–152.

Martinoli C, Derchi LE, Pastorino C et al. Analysis of the echotexture of tendons with US. *Radiology* 1993; **186**: 839–843.

Boal DK, Schwentker EP. Assessment of congenital hip dislocation with real-time ultrasound: a pictorial essay. *Clin Imaging* 1991; **15**(2): 77–90.

Clarke NMP, Clegg J, Al-Chalabi AN. Ultrasound screening of hips at risk for CDH. Failure to reduce the incidence of late cases. *J Bone Joint Surg* (Br) 1989; **71**-B: 9–12.

Graf R, Schuler P. *Sonography of the Infant Hip: An atlas.* Germany, VCH, 1986.

Graf R. Fundamentals of sonographic diagnosis of infant hip dysplasia. *J Pediatr Orthop* 1984; **4**: 735–740.

Harcke HT, Grissom LE. Performing dynamic sonography of the infant hip. *AJR* 1990; **155**: 837–844.

Harcke HT. Screening newborns for developmental dysplasia of the hip: the role of sonography. *AJR* 1994; **162**: 395–397.

Harcke HT, Clarke NMP, Lee MS, Borns PF, MacEwan GD. Examination of the infant hip with real-time sonography. *J Ultrasound Med* 1984; **3**: 131–137.

Jones GT, Schoenecker PL, Dias LS. Developmental hip dysplasia potentiated by inappropriate use of the Pavlik harness. *J Pediatr Orthop* 1992; **12**: 722–726.

Miralles M, Gonzalez G, Pulpeiro JR et al. Sonography of the painful hip in children: 500 consecutive cases. *AJR* 1989; **152**: 579–582.

Poul J, Bajerova J, Skotakova J, Jira I. Selective treatment program for developmental dysplasia of the hip in an epidemiologic prospective study. *J Pediatr Orthop B* 1998; **7**(2): 135–137.

Rosendahl K, Aslaksen A, Lie RT, Markestad T. Reliability of ultrasound in the early diagnosis of developmental dysplasia of the hip. *Pediatr Radiol* 1995; **25**(3): 219–224.

Rosendahl K, Markestad T, Lie RT. Developmental dysplasia of the hip: prevalence based on ultrasound diagnosis. *Pediatr Radiol* 1996; **26**(9): 635–639.

Rosendahl K, Markestad T, Lie RT. Ultrasound screening for developmental dysplasia of the hip in the neonate: the effect on treatment rate and prevalence of late cases. *Pediatrics* 1994; **94**(1): 47–52.

Terjesen T, Bredland T, Berg V. Ultrasound for hip assessment in the newborn. *J Bone Joint Surg (Br)* 1989; **71**-B: 767–773.

Walter RS, Donaldson JS, Davis CL, Shkolnik A, Binns HJ, Carroll NC, Brouillette RT. Ultrasound screening of high-risk infants. A method to increase early detection of congenital dysplasia of the hip. *Am J Dis Child* 1992; **146**(2): 230–234.

Zawin ZK, Hoffer FA, Rand FF, Teele RL. Joint effusion in children with an irritable hip: US diagnosis and aspiration. *Radiology* 1993; **187**: 459–463.

The Hip

Alexander JE, Seibert JJ, Glasier CM et al. High-resolution hip ultrasound in the limping child. *J Clin Ultrasound* 1989; **17**: 19–24.

Alexander JE, Seibert JJ, Aronson J, Williamson SL, Glasier CM, Rodgers AB, Corbitt SL. A protocol of plain radiographs, hip ultrasound, and triple phase bone scans in the evaluation of the painful pediatric hip. *Clin Pediatr Phila* 1988; **27**(4): 175–181.

The Spine

Di Pietro MA. The conus medullaris: normal US findings throughout childhood. *Radiology* 1993; **188**: 149–153.

Garcia CJ, Keller MS. Intraspinal extension of paraspinal masses in infants: detection by sonography. *Pediatr Radiol* 1990; **20**: 437–439.

Kangarloo H, Gold RH, Diament MJ, Boechat MI, Barrett C. High resolution spinal sonography in infants. *AJNR* 1984; **5**: 191–195.

Kawahara H, Andou Y, Takashima S, Takeshita K, Maeda K. Normal development of the spinal cord in neonates and infants seen on ultrasonography. *Neuroradiology* 1987; **29**: 50–52.

Naidich TP, Fernback SK, McLone DG, Scholnik A. Sonography of the caudal spine and back: congenital anomalies in children. *AJNR* 1984; **5**: 221–234.

Naidich TP, Radkowski MA, Britton J. Real-time sonographic display of caudal spinal anomalies. *Neuroradiology* 1986; **28**: 512–527.

Raghavendra BN, Epstein FJ, Pinto RS, Genieser NB, Horii SC. Sonographic diagnosis of diastematomyelia. *J Ultrasound Med* 1988; **7**: 111–113.

Zieger M, Dorr U. Pediatric spinal sonography. Part I: anatomy and examination technique. *Pediatr Radiol* 1988; **18**: 9–13.

Zieger M, Dorr U, Schulz RD. Pediatric spinal sonography. Part II: malformations and mass lesions. *Pediatr Radiol* 1988; **18**: 105–111.

15

COLOUR FLOW, DOPPLER AND POWER MODE IMAGING

Colour flow imaging

Colour flow imaging is a technique which combines the conventional real time grey-scale imaging with a two-dimensional map in which the spatial position of flowing blood is detected, coded and displayed in colour.

The same transducer is used for both grey-scale and colour flow imaging. Blood flow towards the transducer is most commonly coded red and flow away from the transducer most commonly coded blue (Fig. 15.1).

Colour flow imaging is invaluable in clinical practice and has many applications in paediatrics:

- To distinguish a cystic structure from vessels.

- To distinguish a hypoechoic solid mass from a complex fluid collection.

- To assess patency of vessels, e.g. for placement of venous lines and exclusion of thrombus and stenosis.

- For identification of increased blood flow due to inflammation, e.g. appendicitis, epididymitis.

- For identification of decreased or absent blood flow, e.g. when assessing bowel viability in intussusception, establishing a diagnosis of acute testicular torsion.

- To assess developing collateral vessels and varices, e.g. in portal hypertension, and assessing other AV malformations.

Colour flow Doppler imaging

The Doppler principle states that sound reflected off a moving target undergoes a change in frequency. The difference between the transmitted and received frequency is called the Doppler shift frequency.

Colour flow Doppler allows a preselected blood vessel to be assessed regarding its flow characteristics. Sample volumes taken along the ultrasound beam can give a velocity profile of that vessel. There is a range of blood velocities in any one vessel which also vary with time. The blood velocity in arteries has a regular pulsation corresponding to the heartbeat and the velocity in veins often varies with respiration. By measuring the Doppler shift frequency, the Doppler signal can be displayed as a spectral trace or waveform (Figs. 15.2a & b). This can confirm arterial, venous or reversed blood flow and many calculations can be performed on the waveform, e.g. the pulsatility index (PI) and the resistive index (RI).

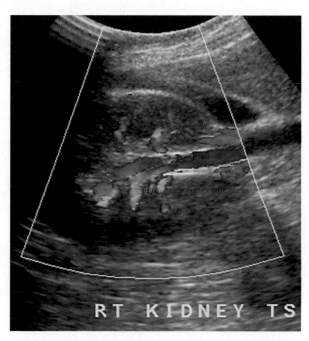

Figure 15.1 — Colour flow imaging of the right kidney in transverse section at the level of the hilum demonstrating arterial (red) and venous (blue) blood flow.

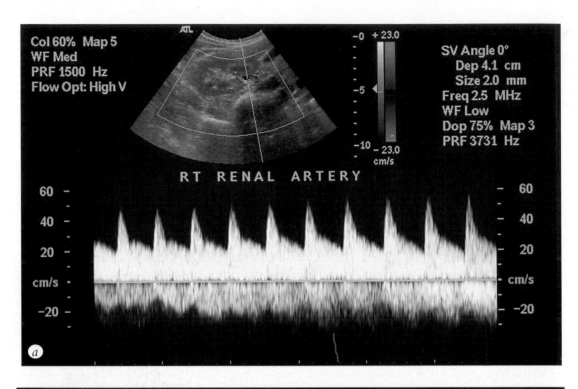

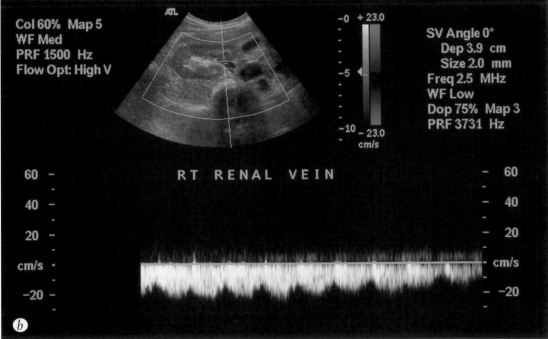

Figure 15.2a & b – Normal renal Doppler waveforms. (a) Spectral display of the right renal artery obtained from a transverse section at the level of the hilum. It demonstrates a prominent systolic peak with a gradual descent and continuous diastolic flow.
(b) Spectral display of the right renal vein obtained from a transverse section at the level of the hilum. It demonstrates continuous blood flow with some respiratory variation.

Power mode

In power mode imaging the presence of blood flow is coded simply as a hue. The luminosity of the colour is arranged to increase with the power of the flow signal without concern for direction (Fig. 15.3).

The power colour scale is therefore continuous, unlike the colour scale in colour flow imaging, and can be chosen according to personal preference.

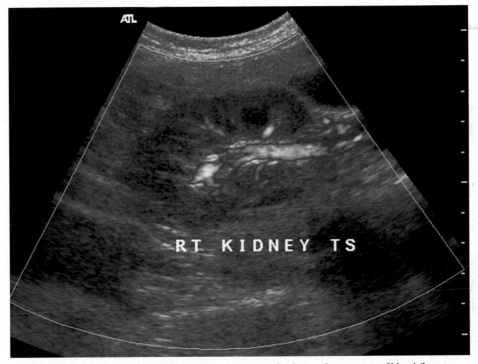

Figure 15.3 — Power mode image of the right kidney in transverse section displaying the presence of blood flow.

INDEX